D0680444

NURSING:
its Hidden Agendas

NURSING:

its Hidden Agendas

Edited by

Moya Jolley

MA (Ed), BSc (Econ), SRN. Dip Ed, RNT, Dip in Nursing (London)
Lecturer, Sociology and Nursing Development,
Institute of Advanced Nursing Education, Royal College
of Nursing, London, UK

and

Gosia Brykczyńska

BSc, BA, RGN, RSCN, Dip PH, Cert Ed, ONC Cert
Lecturer, Nursing Studies, Institute of Advanced
Nursing Education, Royal College of Nursing, London, UK

Edward Arnold
A division of Hodder & Stoughton
LONDON MELBOURNE AUCKLAND

© 1993 MOYA JOLLEY and GOSIA BRYKCZYŃSKA

First published in Great Britain 1993

Distributed in the United States and Canada by
SINGULAR PUBLISHING GROUP, INC.
4284 41st Street
San Diego, California 92105, USA

Library of Congress Cataloguing in Publication Data
Available upon request

Singular ISBN 1–56593 237 4

British Library Cataloguing in Publication Data

Jolley, Moya
  Nursing: Its Hidden Agendas
  I. Title II. Brykczynska, Gosia M.
  610.73

  ISBN 0 340 55726 5

All rights reserved. No part of this publication may be reproduced or transmitted in any
form or by any means, electronically or mechanically, including photocopying, recording
or any information storage or retrieval system, without either prior permission in writing
from the publisher or a licence permitting restricted copying. In the United Kingdom such
licences are issued by the Copyright Licensing Agency: 90 Tottenham Court Road, London
W1P 9HE.

Whilst the advice and information in this book is believed to be true and accurate at
the date of going to press, neither the author nor the publisher can accept any legal
responsibility or liability for any errors or omissions that may be made.

Typeset in 10/11 Times by Hewer Text Composition Services, Edinburgh.
Printed in Great Britain for Edward Arnold, a division of Hodder and
Stoughton Limited, Mill Road, Dunton Green, Sevenoaks, Kent TN13 2YA by
St Edmundsbury Press, Bury St Edmunds, Suffolk and bound by Hartnolls Ltd,
Bodmin, Cornwall. **163668**

BELMONT UNIVERSITY LIBRARY

RT
84.5
.J65
1993

AAY-1288

Preface

Nursing at the present time faces a period of profound change. It will also, potentially, be a period of great opportunity. However, as is well known within the nursing profession itself, change often takes place against a background of criticism and resistance. An inability, sometimes, to come to terms with the need for change, and a clinging to habits and customs of a bygone period not infrequently manifest themselves in both clinical and educational settings. Regular readers of the *Nursing Times* may remember the satirisation of these attitudes in the characterisation of 'Sister Plume'.

This book is an attempt to explore the origins of such attitudes, and their accompanying behaviour patterns; employing historical, psychological, sociological, educational and political perspectives. Attempts are made to trace cause and effect, as well as cross-generational transmission.

The power of hidden agendas in nursing is potentially without limit, unless constructively checked. Contributors have each explored specific aspects, in order to increase understanding of the problems generated, and thus help to facilitate means of constructively addressing them. Each chapter, whilst contributing to the whole, is capable of standing alone as a short study of one chosen perspective on the problems. But ideally this is a book which should be read as a whole in order meaningfully to address this multi-faceted phenomenon.

If the progress of nursing is to move forward smoothly into the twenty-first century, it can no longer afford to enshrine within its professional ethos elements inimical to that progression.

Despite the problems alluded to above, there appears to be a dearth of material relevant to the British context which addresses this subject. Bearing in mind the juncture in its history that nursing in this country has now reached, it seems appropriate that a critical, in-depth exploration of this powerful, and potentially negative, force in nursing should now be attempted.

London
August 1992

Moya Jolley
Gosia Brykczyńska

Acknowledgements

The editors would like to extend their grateful thanks to all the contributors to this book. Without their enthusiastic commitment, and great generosity in time and energy, its production would not have been possible. Our thanks go to Dr Krauss for writing the foreword; also to Miss Maria Bnińska, Ms Jill Waites, and the Rev. Mervyn Pendleton for assisting in manuscript preparation. Appreciation and thanks also go to Ms Helen Thomas, Assistant Librarian in the Library of Nursing at the Royal College of Nursing for her great support and meticulous care in the checking and preparation of references. We would also like to thank Mrs Jean Smith who continued to provide help and support throughout the period of manuscript preparation. Lastly, our thanks go to Mrs Nancy Loffler for her unfailing help and enthusiasm in developing this book.

Contents

Preface   v

Acknowledgements   vii

List of contributors   x

1 Out of the past
   Moya Jolley   1
2 The psychology of attitudes and values
   Julia Mingay   21
3 A sociologist's view: the handmaiden's theory
   Abigayl Perry   43
4 Hidden curricula in nursing education
   Stella Pendleton   80
5 Political influences in nursing
   Amanda Tattam and *Marjorie Thompson*   107
6 Nursing Values: nightmares and nonsense
   Gosia Brykczyńska   131
7 Closing thoughts on hidden agendas – an epilogue
   Caroline Cox   159

Index   173

List of contributors

Gosia Brykczyńska, BSc, BA, RGN, RSCN, Dip PH, Cert Ed, ONC Cert
Lecturer, Nursing Studies, Institute of Advanced Nursing Education, Royal
College of Nursing, London

Caroline Cox (Baroness Cox of Queensbury), MSc(Econ), BSc(Soc), RGN
Deputy Speaker, House of Lords

Moya Jolley, MA(Ed), BSc(Econ), SRN. Dip Ed, RNT, Dip in Nursing (London) Lecturer, Sociology and Nursing Development, Institute of Advanced
Nursing Education, Royal College of Nursing, London

Julia Mingay, MSc, RGN, RMN, RNT, RCNT, Dip Nursing, Cert in Counselling. Lecturer, Psychology and Education Studies, Institute of Advanced
Nursing Education, Royal College of Nursing, London

Stella Pendleton, MA(Ed), BH(Hons), RGN, RSCN, RM, Dip Nursing
(London), MTD Vice Principal, Institute of Advanced Nursing Education,
Royal College of Nursing, London

Abigayl Perry, BSc Hon(Soc), MSc(Econ), RGN, FETC
Freelance lecturer and writer

Amanda Tattam, RGN (Melbourne)
Reporter, Nursing Times

Marjorie Thompson, BSc(Hons), MSc(Econ)
Advisor, Department of Policy and Practice, Royal College of Nursing and
Chairperson, Campaign for Nuclear Disarmament

1 Out of the past

You are not here to think Nurse

(Anon)

An American nurse journalist writing of socialisation within a profession commented that

> If the heritage of nursing is considered to be an important vehicle for professional socialization, guidance for the present should be based on lessons from the past . . . Many current norms of practice and professional behaviour are perpetuated and enacted without a full understanding of their emergence in history, or their relevance for today's practice.
>
> (Wheeler, 1985)

Though Wheeler was writing of the North American context, her comments are equally applicable to the British situation. This chapter seeks to provide a very brief background sketch of where nursing has come from; identifying influences which have contributed to its tradition, structure, relationships, and development, (the seedbed of elements constituting the modern hidden agenda) which will then be addressed in depth in the chapters that follow. It is not intended to be definitive, or to include a whole range of potentially relevant data, but hopefully to stimulate the reader's interest to explore further in to his/her professional past.

Modern nursing, as it is currently conceived to be, was born in the second half of the nineteenth-century. Institutions and professions reflect, within their own structures, the society in which they have their being; including prevailing norms, attitudes, beliefs and values. Early pioneers in nursing have been frequently, and occasionally bitterly, criticised for their part in formulating and transmitting a tradition, in many of its aspects now seen to be inimical to professional development and progress in nursing in the modern era. Like Tevye in 'Fiddler on the Roof' tradition has sometimes been thought to be 'the most important thing in life'.

However, to endeavour to attain any understanding of how this tradition, in its multiplicity of facets and influences, came to be shaped and moulded in the way that it did, it is necessary to consider in a little detail the social structure and cultural context of the period. Political and economic, as well as social and environmental factors, exerted powerful influences then, as they continue to do in the present era, and nursing in common with most other occupations is not immune to these.

The nineteenth century is sometimes referred to by historians as a century of progress, and as a century of scientific discovery. The industrial revolution was still in progress; though the term 'revolution' here could be seen as something of a misnomer, as violent and bloody change so often associated with that term was not a dominant feature; indeed the process of industrial change was fairly slow. However, the factory system continued to develop as new industrial technology was introduced, despite employers' fears of increasing financial costs, and employees' fears of 'wage slavery'.

The extention of industry was accompanied by the uncontrolled growth of towns, which in turn spawned housing, sanitary and health problems of some magnitude. These difficulties were further exacerbated by a marked population growth through the period. In 1801 the census recorded a population of 9,000,000. This doubled by 1851 and was to double again by 1901. It was essentially a young population, where in 1850 75 per cent were under the age of 45 years. Married persons constituted 36 per cent and single persons 60 per cent of the overall population.

This period also saw the beginnings of women's emancipation and, despite opposition from landed interests, the extention of the franchise in 1832 to the rising entrepreneurial wealthy middle class merchants and manufacturers. Further reform acts were to follow which would eventually enfranchise the whole of the male population. The right to vote was not extended to women however, before a long, bitter and sometimes violent struggle had ensued, spanning several decades, before its final achievement early in the twentieth century.

Queen Victoria ascended the throne in 1837, and the period following, until her death in 1901, is often referred to as the 'Victorian era'; frequently associated in the popular mind with images of wealth, progress, extention of Empire, invention, exploration, and also with a cluster of dominant norms, attitudes, values and beliefs, sometimes referred to collectively as 'Victorianism'. The period was also linked to accusations of complacency, narrow mindedness, prudery, dullness, and resistance to social change. All these elements played a significant part in the early shaping of nursing, and will be referred to again later in this chapter and others.

The Victorian era was not, however, a period of uniform prosperity. Prior to the repeal of the Corn Laws in 1847 there was much rural poverty, with labourers starving, minimum wages fixed in most counties, and considerable unrest. The unrest, sporadic violence and the Chartist movement caused unease among the ruling classes who, mindful of recent events in Europe, feared revolution. Repeal did not, however, bring agricultural ruin as had been feared by some, and the three decades that followed saw increasing prosperity and the more extensive adoption of improved methods of cultivation first introduced a century earlier.

Despite these improvements though, the drift from the land began among the rural working class, and by 1881 there were 100,000 fewer farm labourers. The last quarter of the nineteenth century showed a reverse trend in agriculture, with depression replacing prosperity. Poor harvests, outbreaks of cattle disease, as well as increasing competition from abroad meant mounting losses for farmers, many of whom became bankrupt. Reduced wages drove many farm labourers to seek employment in towns, and much land went out of cultivation. The forces of industrial and agricultural change brought about an increase in those seeking employment in an urban setting. Factories had been, and were still being organised on a principle of *laissez-faire*, and were subject to few regulations. The guiding principle was profit making for the factory owners, and health and safety of employees was not a prime consideration. Women and children were employed in considerable numbers as they were generally cheaper than male labour, while conditions of child labour were often little short of slavery. Wages were low, and working hours were long, with methods of coercion amounting to cruelty sometimes employed.

A series of Factory Acts, designed to ameliorate the worst aspects of the system were enacted, the first effective piece of legislation being passed in 1833. Resistance inevitably arose, with protests that industry would be adversely affected by restricting child labour. Resentment of what was viewed as State interference was much in evidence, as was the so-called pseudo-philanthropy that suggested that work could only be provided on existing terms, and was therefore preferable for all concerned. Southgate (1965) draws attention to perhaps somewhat unexpected opposition to factory legislation from the Women's Rights movement. He comments:

> Women of the upper and middle classes resented their exclusion from the franchise and from the learned professions, and some who were agitating for the removal of these disabilities saw in the limitations imposed on women's work in factories further examples of injustice to their sex.

As mentioned earlier, growth of the factory system was also accompanied by unregulated urban development. Poor housing, overcrowding, defective sewage and refuse disposal systems, as well as contaminated water, adulterated food, and a generally low standard of hygiene all contributed to epidemics at frequent intervals. John Simon, later to become medical officer to the General Board of Health, commented that 'it was no uncommon thing, in a room 12 feet square or less, to find three to five families styed together . . . in the promiscuous intimacy of cattle'.

In 1842 Edwin Chadwick, sometimes known as the 'father of English Sanitation', published his famous 'Survey into the Sanitary Condition of the People' (Briggs, 1983). This has been described as the death blow to the 'let things alone' party. Chadwick was an untiring worker for the setting up of a Sanitary Commission, which he was eventually successful in establishing, leading on to the first Public Health Act 1848 (adoptive only). Other individuals in the field also worked tirelessly to improve standards of health, hygiene and sanitation, including Dr Thomas Southwood Smith, founder of the 'Health of Towns Association' and the aforementioned Dr John Simon who was influential in the institution of sanitary inspectors, and the introduction of measures to improve drainage, housing, and other related ills of the time. However, the general tenor of public feeling was not particularly favourable to the efforts of such reformers, as was reflected in a comment in *The Times* newspaper of the period 'we prefer to take our chance of Cholera and the rest rather than be bullied into health' (Briggs, 1983). Progress was slow, but further epidemics of cholera, and outbreaks of diphtheria, smallpox and typhus ensured eventual victory for the reformers with the passing of the great Public Health Act of 1875.

Poverty among both the rural and urban working classes remained a problem throughout the Victorian era. A Royal Commission to study the workings of the Poor Law was set up in 1832, resulting in the Poor Law Amendment Act of 1834. The Act was what would now probably be described as draconian, producing harsh changes which undoubtedly must have inflicted considerable suffering upon the poor. Workhouses were designed to be places of dread, where the principle of 'less eligibility' ensured the grimmest of conditions for the luckless inmates. Expenditure on relief to the poor was reduced by harsh application of the provisions of the Act, but poverty was not reduced thereby, nor employment found for those willing to work. The poor continued to live in fear of unemployment, sickness and old age until well into the twentieth century, when more humane and positive approaches were made in addressing the underlying causes of poverty.

The middle period of the Victorian era was not, as indicated above, one sympathetic to the disadvantaged or the weaker members of society. It was a period described by Briggs (1983) as being 'proud, confident and prosperous'. England was the richest country in the world. There was a degree of social stability, even though tensions lurked below the surface. Economic, technological and scientific development was proceeding apace, and the concept of self-help, as epitomised in the book of the same title by Samuel Smiles published in 1850, was lauded. The Victorians valued such qualities as thrift, hard work, abstinence, strength of character and respectability.

Throughout the period Britain was governed mainly by a landed aristocracy, and social class divisions were fairly rigid. Ascribed status carried more weight than did achieved position, and social mobility was limited.

As the century passed its mid-point and industrial progress gave rise to a new power, that of the industrial middle class, there also arose new needs in terms of a more highly skilled workforce. Education therefore became an issue, giving rise to opposing viewpoints concerning the need for a more literate and numerate working class. The Church of England and the Non-Conformist Church, realising the increasing need for literacy among the poorer sections of the population sought to remedy the situation. Regrettably rival bodies were set up in the form of the Church of England National Society and the Non-Conformist British and Foreign Schools Society which opposed and frustrated Government efforts to establish a national system of schooling. Despite these problems the Forster Education Act was passed in 1870, ensuring non-denominational, compulsory education in the basic subjects of reading, writing and arithmetic to the age of 10 years for all children. This was raised to 11 years in 1893 and to 12 years in 1899. Education at this point in time was selective in content and structured according to social class position. Control of education was firmly in the hands of the ruling class, who viewed education for the working classes, if they did not actually oppose it, as enabling them to become 'efficient machine minders'. Rudimentary education including religious instruction was seen as a means of 'gentleing the masses'.

As the century progressed trade unionism began to develop from its rather tentative beginnings earlier in the period. Unionism in the 1850s and 1860s developed first among skilled workers, but the last quarter of the century saw it being extended to the unskilled also, for example in Ben Tillett's Tea Workers and General Labourers Union, and the Gas Workers Union of Joseph Arch. Various acts of Parliament sought both to regulate activities and protect union funds. However, it was not until the twentieth century that trades union power began to assume significant proportions.

The second half of the nineteenth-century witnessed a developing social consciousness. There were indications of a growing religious tolerance, and evangelicalism and non-conformism grew. In the 1850s Oxford and Cambridge Universities began to admit non-conformists. Those of the Jewish faith were enabled to become members of Parliament, and greater freedom was extended to Roman Catholics. In 1878 William Booth founded the Salvation Army, bringing a practical Christianity initially to the east end of London, and thereafter to wider spheres of influence (Rundle, 1973).

The triumphs of commerce and industry however, along with the growing extremes of wealth and poverty, began to be questioned. The poet Matthew Arnold complained of 'this strange disease of modern life with its sick hurry, its divided aims' (Briggs, 1983) – a complaint which could perhaps be reiterated today.

There was no dearth of great social reformers during this period, one of the greatest perhaps being the Earl of Shaftesbury. Pioneers existed in many fields, including workhouse and prison reform, higher education, female emancipation, maternity and child care, and mental health, to mention but a few areas of activity. The progress of all these areas tended to be slow. Trevelyan described the period as being a liberal, outspoken age, with social customs and economic circumstances always in movement, changing, yet not completely, and not all at once (Trevelyan, 1946). Escott saw 'old lines of demarcation' being obliterated, 'ancient landmarks of thought and faith removed . . . The idols which were revered but a little time ago have been destroyed' (Briggs, 1983).

Disquiet remained in many quarters of Victorian society. Writers such as John Stuart Mill, and novelists such as Charles Dickens raised social questions that demanded to be addressed. The second half of the century saw the creation of the first socialist organisation in Britain, the Democratic Federation of Henry Hyndman in 1861. Later a group of middle class intellectuals were to form the Fabian Society in 1884, to be followed by the formation of the Independent Labour Party in 1893. This in turn developed into the Labour Party at the turn of the century, representing the working class voice at Parliamentary level; one day to challenge successfully the domination of both the Liberal and Conservative Parties.

The call to public service was an increasingly powerful force as the Victorian era progressed. It manifested itself in the work of individual reformers, often upper middle-class women, some of whom were 'in flight from the drawing room'. It showed itself in the work of voluntary organisations and pressure groups. Gladstone's 'rule of ought' where duty was seen to be more important than personal desires, lay at the heart of this aspect of Victorian behaviour. Briggs (1983) comments that the shrine of the 'rule of ought' was the home.

In Victorian society the family was viewed as the cornerstone; the home was venerated and women were placed on a pedestal. The home was seen as a retreat and protection from society, as illustrated in this comment from Ruskin in 1865:

> This is the true nature of home – it is the place of PEACE; the shelter, not only from all injury, but from all terror, doubt and division. In so far as it is not this, it is not home; so far as the anxieties of the outer life penetrate into it, and the inconsistently minded, unloved, or hostile society of the outer world is allowed by either husband or wife to cross the threshold it ceases to be home . . .
>
> (Thrift and Williams, 1987)

The 'perfect lady', so beloved of the Victorians, was in reality a middle-class ideal.

> Her status was totally dependent upon the economic position of her father, and then her husband. In her most perfect form the lady combined total sexual innocence, conspicuous consumption and the worship of the family hearth.
>
> (Vicinus, 1972)

This somewhat narrow definition was at some distance from the reality experienced by many women of the period. Delamont and Duffin comment that this 'perfect lady' image rendered middle-class women more and more useless. Conspicuous consumption and leisured existence were, in themselves, status symbols of family affluence and success. This complete uselessness led to a belief in the incapability of such women, and their need to be prohibited from serious participation in society (Delamont and Duffin, 1978). The deification of motherhood also served to keep such women out of mainstream social activity.

The Victorian woman has also been viewed as a

> doll-like, bread and butter miss, swooning on a sofa, or a sickly mother dying under the strain of a dozen births, or a straight-laced, thin-lipped middle class prude hidden in an over-ornamented pyramid of bombazine, who bullied her servants and looked down her nose at her neighbours.
>
> (Crow, 1971)

The writer goes on to point out that these stereotypes were not representative of all women of the period, reminding his readers that women were also factory workers, governesses, sweated labourers, writers and reformers. As with so many stereotypes the 'perfect lady' and the 'Victorian woman' were neither perfect nor typical.

The position and role of women in Victorian society constituted one of the most important topics through the period. There were many conflicting view-points surrounding the issues. In 1869 John Stuart Mill wrote on the

'Subjection of Women'. His view of marriage as a partnership between those of intellectual and emotional equality was seen as an aberration; while the view of Ruskin that women were 'flowers to be plucked' tended to be closer to the accepted norm. The novels of Trollope and the Brontës reflect the image of the middle-class Victorian woman, while Dickens often portrayed graphically the role and position of women of the lower social classes. Elizabeth Garrett Anderson, the first British woman physician and herself a middle-class woman, wrote in 1850:

> I was a young woman living at home with nothing to do in what authors call 'comfortable circumstances'. But I was wicked enough not to be comfortable. I was full of energy and vigour, and with the discontent which goes with unemployed activities.
>
> (Manton, 1965)

The world of the Victorian woman was a man-made world. Women's activities were, and had always been seen in relation to those of men, rather than independently. Tradition, custom, scientific practice, and law, all played a part in prescribing the limits of her activities. 'The role of men never became the soul-searching matter in the same way as did that of women' (Lewis, 1984). Women's education was largely seen as preparation for future roles as wives and mothers. Education was to develop their 'natural' submission to authority, and to encourage their maternal instinct. They were not expected to develop personal opinions beyond the trivial. Indeed one writer on women's etiquette suggested that a woman's highest duty was to 'suffer and be still' (Vicinus, 1972). Interestingly the writer was a woman.

The unmarried woman was seen as a failure. Satirised and criticised, the spinster frequently experienced both financial and psycho-social difficulties resulting directly from the force of social norms and attitudes of the time.

Although Victorian women were not always passive and accepting of their position in society, they faced formidable problems in terms of breaking free of the stereotypical 'ideal woman' image. Society exerted powerful control by means of its demand for 'respectability', and its sanctions on deviance from the accepted norms of female behaviour.

This dominant stereotype held sway even among working class women, where its attainment was virtually impossible '"Grundyism" was a powerful force in the service of duty over passion, and obedience over independence,' (Vicinus, 1972). Female adultery was seen as threatening the very fabric of society. A 'fallen woman' in the family meant dire consequences in terms of loss of respectability, if not also employment.

As the century progressed however, the sphere of moral and social activity began to widen. Matters for debate in society now included marriage laws, job opportunities, education and female emigration. Marriage, however, continued to confer greater status than spinsterhood, and continued to be the life expectation of the majority of women. For most working-class women it was little short of a practical necessity.

Middle-class wives were expected to remain in the home, though charity work was seen as an acceptable outlet for frustrated energies. Even here though an excessive zeal tended to be frowned upon. Magazines and journals designed for a female readership reflected, and furthered, the prevailing social norms and expectations as they related to women. The position could be summed up in a portion of Tennyson's poem 'The Princess':

> Man for the field, woman for the hearth,
> Man for the sword and for the needle she;
> Man with the head and woman with the heart,
> Man to command and woman to obey.
>
> (Tennyson, 1953)

A woman was expected to be chaste prior to marriage, and to desire nothing more than to be the helpmeet of her husband. She was required to be righteous, sympathetic, but above all submissive. A 'married woman' indicated a woman who had no existence in common law apart from her husband. She had no legal right to property, could not give testimony in court, and had no legal right to her children. In matters of divorce, while adultery was the only cause needed when sought by a husband, a wife had to prove an additional charge of either cruelty, desertion, bigamy, incest, rape, sodomy, or bestiality (Branca, 1975).

Once married, continuous child-bearing and the raising of large families was the norm, though the 1890s saw a slow reduction in family size, starting among the upper classes. With the home a potential prison, her role rigidly circumscribed with limited outlet for energy or talent, it is perhaps not surprising that there appeared to be what some historians regard as an 'explosion' of female illness in the second half of the nineteenth century. Sometimes referred to as a 'flight into illness' (Delamont and Duffin, 1978).

Much of this illness appears to have emanated from the middle-class level of society, where hypochondria, often exacerbated by enforced inactivity, was validated by the medical profession of the time. Female physiological function was often viewed by doctors as pathological. Puberty and menstruation were seen in the *Anthropological Review* of 1869

> as an 'affliction' producing 'languor' and depression which disqualify them for thought or action and render it extremely doubtful how far they can be considered responsible beings while the crisis lasts.
>
> (Delamont and Duffin, 1978)

Of pregnancy it was said that it was 'nervous force that goes astray in every direction' (Delamont and Duffin, 1978). Henry Maudsley, writing in the Fortnightly Review of 1874, suggested that

> women could never hope to equal masculine accomplishments, because their physiology acts as a handicap, body and mind being for one quarter of each month during the best years of life . . . more or less sick and unfit for hard work.
>
> (Vicinus, 1972)

It has been suggested that medicine both reflects and reinforces the dominant beliefs and values of any one particular period, and plays a part in shaping roles and options, thereby acting as a social force in society, in addition to its manifest function of healing. In thus reinforcing dominant social values it contributes to the conservation of the socio-economic status quo. Chapter 3 will address in depth the power of sociological factors as they have influenced health care through the twentieth century, and thereby the activity of nursing.

In a rapidly changing social context such as the later Victorian period represents, both science and medicine were invoked to endeavour to justify gender inequalities. Darwinistic Victorian scientists suggested that female evolution was either incomplete, or arrested earlier than the male. This was believed to be in order to permit conservation of energy for child-bearing. Many doctors of the time believed that women's intellectual activities should be curbed to protect their prime function of reproduction, and most female ailments were ascribed to uterine malfunction (Lewis, 1984).

The coercive power of religious tradition, now in decline, was replaced by that of medicine and science. Little wonder that many medical men fiercely resisted the entrance of women into the medical profession. Dr Tilt in the Lancet in 1869 (Delamont and Duffin, 1978) described them in a somewhat ungentlemanly way as 'sexless philosophers' and 'epicene agitators'. Delamont and Duffin (1978) point out that medical theorists of the time provided a view of women, in terms of health, that varied according to social class position. Middle-class women were shown as being delicate and weak, but working-class women were seen as 'sickening', and a health hazard, undermining the fitness of the race via the production of numerous inferior off-spring. It is hardly necessary to state that the reality was somewhat different.

The deeper underlying factor informing many of the foregoing attitudes was male fear of an erosion of dominance, and possible competition from women in both social and economic spheres. They would perhaps have preferred Virginia Woolf's later somewhat cynical description of women's role: 'Women have served all these centuries as looking glasses possessing the magic and delicious power of reflecting the figure of man at twice its natural size' (Woolf, 1929). History has demonstrated that their fear was not without foundation!

By the 1880s the role of the 'perfect lady' was being challenged. Job opportunities were expanding, and legal restrictions relating to women were slowly being removed. Educational opportunities beyond the elementary level were opening up, and by the turn of the century a number of universities were accepting women to their degree courses. These reforms, together with the activities of the Women's Suffrage movement, and the activities of individuals prepared to accept rejection and isolation in order to initiate reforms and change attitudes, all contributed to a breakdown in hypocrisy and rigidity as it related to gender issues in Victorian society.

Although it must have seemed slow and tortuous to many women at the time, social change was taking place, though several more decades would be needed before women achieved the aims of the Suffrage movement, improved their economic positions radically, or were freely able to pursue professional careers. However, as Boyd points out, women reformers by placing women's issues in a separate category were vulnerable to the criticism of being concerned only with that, and not wider society, thus enhancing existing male prejudices

(Boyd, 1982)

Although attitudes were now showing indications of change staying single was still seen to be a 'deliberate revolt against the prescribed feminine role' (Lewis, 1984). However, independent women were now being portrayed in literature (usually a fairly reliable reflection of the current social scene) as heroines for the first time. Even so, as Lewis points out,

the framework formed by theories of sexual differences imposed upon women formed part of the social background and context within which women had to work, both feminist and non-feminist.

Women were still struggling to break free from the 'Angel in the Home' image of Coventry Patmore.

As indicated earlier, the nineteenth century though a period of rapid change and progress on many fronts, was also a period that produced a multiplicity of social and humanitarian problems. Not the least of these was the care of the sick. In the early part of the period such institutional nursing as there was got carried out either by nuns whose motivation was primarily religious, or by women from what were referred to collectively as the 'lower orders'. The second type, as is well known, has been immortalised by Charles Dickens in his characters of Sairy Gamp and Betsy Prigg. These images, as Bedford Fenwick was to remark,

clothed in bombazine and redolent of gin, were by no means creatures of his own imagination, but distinct types . . . of women actually in existence, and who had stamped the profession of Nursing with utter contempt and ridicule, instilling into the minds of the public an intrinsic antipathy to hospitals, infirmaries and workhouses, and which will take the combined forces of knowledge, sympathy and refinement, years to eradicate.

(Bedford Fenwick, 1888)

Whittaker and Oleson (1964) suggest that 'at the time of the Crimean war the world of nursing in Europe was straining to evolve from the province of the sacred on the one hand, and from the profane on the other'. They suggest that Florence Nightingale rescued nursing from the latter category. The image of the nurse was transformed for ever following her work in the Crimea, investing her personally with the mantle of a national heroine, and ensuring that from that time nursing bore her image rather than that of Gamp. This served as a status elevator for nursing in a period when such seemingly heroic activities appealed to certain aspects of the dominant value system.

Florence Nightingale herself was a woman well-educated by the standards of the time, who had few illusions about the difficulties faced by her own sex in Victorian society. In 1852, she wrote 'Why have women passion, intellect, moral activity – these three – and a place in society where no one of these three can be exercised?' She goes on, speaking of passions, to say that:

'In conventional society which men have made for women, and women have accepted, they MUST have none, they MUST act the farce of hypocrisy . . .'. Later she writes of 'cold, conventional oppressive atmospheres where satisfaction of intellect, passion and moral activity cannot be satisfied'. She complains that women 'cannot live in the light of intellect. Society forbids it.

Those conventional frivolities which are called "duties" forbid it'. (Nightingale, 1979). A little later she comments, perhaps a little cynically, 'that man and woman have an equality of duties and rights is accepted by woman even less than by man'.

However, the legend of Nightingale, 'the lady with the lamp', was carefully tuned to what were deemed to be culturally desirable feminine attributes; and so the picture of the frail, dedicated, saintly Crimean heroine emerged. The reality, as many modern writers on Nightingale indicate, was somewhat different, revealing a strong, ruthless, manipulative, aggressive, and at times neurotic personality (Smith, 1982). These less desirable traits (at least by nineteenth century standards) were largely ignored, and the popular image was in harmony with the age of Romanticism and Humanitarianism. The Victorian milieu was receptive to the values represented by Nightingale.

In many respects, however, she defied and refused to enact in her own life the role demanded of her as an upper middle-class woman of her era. Whittaker and Oleson (1964) point out that 'she stretched the very boundaries of 19th century womanhood to encompass feats hitherto unknown for genteel females'.

Nursing prior to the Nightingale reforms was at a low ebb, and hospitals often insanitary and dangerous places. They were mostly for the poor; the rich and influential members of society, usually being nursed by servants at home, were unaffected by the evils that existed, and therefore for the most part indifferent to them.

In order to establish secular nursing, as Bullough and Bullough (1979) point out, it was necessary not only to convince hospital administrators and physicians that good nursing care was important, the public had also to be convinced. More importantly women themselves had to believe that nursing was a vital and important job worthy of their talents, and that there was nothing disgraceful about becoming a nurse.

The scientific and medical progress extant through the period was to work in favour of nursing reform. As advances were made in medicine and bacteriology, and as the introduction of anaesthesia opened the way to advances in surgery, many physicians began to recognise the need for higher standards of care than had existed hitherto.

The story of the establishment of the first nurse training school, financed by the Nightingale Fund from money donated by a grateful nation, is well known and does not need to be repeated here. However, early historical accounts have tended to be somewhat uncritical, not to say adulatory, and it has been left to modern historians, some of them nurses themselves, to seek closer approximations to the truth.

Baly suggests that, contrary to popular perception, Nightingale did not return from the Crimea intent immediately on setting about the reform of nursing, and indeed regarded the Fund as 'a millstone round her neck' (Baly, 1986). Prince, writing in 1984, also draws attention to the problems of the Nightingale School during its early years. These were related both to administrative incompetence, as well as to the failure to provide adequate teaching, and the work overload experienced by probationers. By 1873 Nightingale could write, as she did to Henry Bonham-Carter, that 'our School is not a training school, it is taking half the hospital's work'. In an earlier letter to the same correspondent, she had stated 'We must begin now, all over again, if we don't we are ruined' (Woodham-Smith, 1950).

Carter (1939) suggests that Nightingale wished to restore to nursing the prestige it once had under the religious orders. Her idea of the 'perfect nurse' embraced a concept of triple motivation: natural, intellectual and religious. However, the whole idea of a training school for nurses was a novel one in Britain at the time, and was viewed with a degree of hostility by some members of the medical profession, who felt that trained nurses might encroach, or even challenge, their authority.

The prestige of Nightingale ensured that the school was established despite such opposition, and it opened on 9 July 1860. Rules and regulations had been drawn up by Nightingale, and the early probationers entered a world strictly regulated and protected. The Nurses Home was an integral part of this protective system. They worked long hours, and experienced what, by modern standards, was a harsh discipline. Flirtation was punished by dismissal, and marriage meant termination of employment. The School was structured along social class lines, candidates being admitted either as probationers or as special probationers who were 'of higher social standing', and paid for the training they received.

> The daily life of the Nightingale Probationers in the early years provided for attic cubicles in dreary hospital living quarters located in a 'rough and squalid neighbourhood', irregular lecturers, antiquated medical books, and practice on a dummy in a rudimentary laboratory.
>
> (Seymer, 1960)

That things did not go well for the Nightingale School in its early days was glossed over by early historians. Nevertheless records indicate that only approximately 60% of probationers completed their courses. Many were dismissed either for misconduct or due to illness. As for being a 'School for Matrons', as Baly points out, in the first ten years it produced only two superintendents (Baly, 1986).

Both military and religious influences mingled in Nightingale's approach to nursing reform. Palmer suggests that the future image was in fact cast during the Crimean war period. A relationship to medicine and hospital administration was established that placed nursing below both (Palmer, 1983).

Nightingale, though a far-seeing and forward-thinking woman, was also a child of her age. She was highly conscious of social class divisions, coming herself from the untitled aristocracy. Her concept of the ordinary nurse was that of a member of the servant class. She suggested living conditions and working hours similar to those of servants in a typical upper middle-class household. The uniform bore a strong resemblance to that of domestic servants of the period. The qualities of a good nurse she envisaged as 'restraint, discipline and obedience'.

> She should carry out the orders of the doctors in a suitably humble and deferential way. She should obey to the letter the requirements of the matron and the sister.
>
> (Davies, 1977)

Nightingale did not envisage 'ladies' in any other role than that of matron, and indeed seemed uneasy regarding their entry into nurse training.

> As regards ladies . . . difficulties attend their admission; yet their eventual admixture to a certain extent in the work is an important feature of it. Obedience, discipline, self-control, work understood as work, hospital service as implying masters, civil and medical, and a mistress, what service means, and abnegation of self, are things not always easy to be learnt, understood and faithfully acted upon by ladies . . . their dismissal . . . must always be more troublesome, if not more difficult than that of other nurses.
>
> (Nightingale, 1858)

She was not alone in her thinking here. Elizabeth Garrett Anderson, commenting on the introduction of lady volunteers into nursing staffs of both King's College and University College Hospitals, states:

> A lady who, with very little training, does hospital nursing in a first rate way, is 'a priori' likely to be able to do much more difficult things; and the question is whether it is desirable, for the sake of saving money to the hospital, to limit her permanently to work of so subordinate a character . . . Admirably as ladies can nurse, the actual work of nursing is not much more appropriate to them than of cooking and dusting in their own homes.
>
> (Garrett, 1867).

Palmer comments that

> By the time nursing was organised into a system of training, the image of the nurse – subordinate, servile, domestic, humble, self-sacrificing, and not too learned – was inculcated into society.
>
> (Palmer, 1983)

It is interesting to note that such an image fitted well, in many aspects, into the Victorian image of the 'ideal woman'. Nursing came to be seen as a 'safe sacrifice' for virtuous and dedicated women. It was not to break free of this image for many decades, and half a century later a nurse academic could write:

Nursing has been secularised, but it has in its bones nearly 2,000 years of submission to religious order. The urge to obey, to kiss the rod, with its obverse the love of power, are not absent in a modern world, and nursing, especially institutional nursing, tends still to be a refuge, conscious or unconscious, for the naturally submissive.

(Carter, 1939)

It could be added that it was not only monastic influences at work here, but social and gender influences of the Victorian era, given an extended lease of life within an occupation tentatively seeking an identity, yet fearful of change.

Some historians argue that these characteristics of deference and obedience were eminently practical, and made reasonable sense AT THE TIME. Matrons of the period encouraged, and sought to reinforce, both in their own areas of responsibility and in nursing journals of the time, such patterns of behaviour in their nurses.

Miss Mollett, a London Matron, writing in the *Nursing Record* of 1888 states:

No lesson is harder to learn for a new nurse than that of discipline – the subordination of her will unquestioningly to that of another . . . she must bend under a law which is by no means always a law of love; never ask 'why', and as seldom as possible 'how'; be content to bear unmerited blame without murmuring, to be scolded for mistakes that were made in all good faith; she must not be surprised to find herself vehemently repressed if she ventures on the faintest suggestion, and generally, especially if she is at all forward or clever she will be 'put in her right place'.

She has the grace to admit that 'when power rests in the hands of unsuitable people it undoubtedly degenerates from proper discipline into very intolerable petty tyranny'.

She continues at some length in a similar exhortatory vein; one paragraph must stand as representative of an article of some considerable length.

Among all the good qualities which a perfect nurse should possess, a little of that 'courage of endurance', that spirit of self-sacrifice, which was so important a point with the old religious sisters, would not be a bad thing. Cheerful obedience to discipline, the idea of accepting restraint in any spirit but a hostile one, loyalty to superiors, faithful submission to subordination are the very rarest virtues among them. Yet it is the spirit of self-sacrificing loyalty that leads to the highest and truest discipline . . . that remains loyally silent over its own wrongs, and punctilious to a fault in the fulfillment of its duties.

She ends this rather awesome account by commenting that 'no life is more hard to live nobly than a life of loyal servitude'. Articles of a similar tenor appear in much of the nursing literature of the time. It should be borne in mind also, however, as Davies notes, that the deferential nurse as envisaged by Nightingale was in no way a threat to the doctor or an encroachment on his territory. A stress on docility and discipline, drawn from military and religious organizations . . . served to attract middle class recruits, and represented a very necessary attack on the prevailing image of the nurse.

(Davies, 1977)

Viewed in terms of the needs of nineteenth-century nursing, such an argument can be seen to be valid. What gave rise to problems in the decades that followed was the determined maintenance of, and clinging to, a tradition and image, parts of which, as the nineteenth century progressed, were to become increasingly non-viable. Qualities once lauded, and the attitudes engendered in their development, could become not only inappropriate and undesirable, but dangerous and obstructive. Later chapters will explore these issues.

One of Nightingale's other strategies in launching her reform was to combine the position of matron with that of head of the training school. The subordination of training to the service needs of the hospital was then laid down, to be a source of trial and conflict far into the future. Nightingale, emphasised the importance of 'character development' in nurses, rather than 'education', and was resistant to written examinations as a test of nursing quality.

'No living thing can less lend itself to a formula than nursing. Nursing has to nurse living bodies and spirits. It must be sympathetic. It cannot be tested by public examination, though it may be tested by current supervision.'

(Rathbone, 1890)

It should be borne in mind that the founding of the Nightingale School antedated mass education for all, and that problems of illiteracy were a feature of the period.

As is well known, a structural hierarchy developed in the early foundation period of nursing reform. Davies comments that

a division of labour built in firm differences of status and power, which distinguished the 'ordinary probationer' from the 'lady pupils'. It was the latter who were to be groomed for posts as matrons

(Davies, 1977)

Thus the early division within the profession of elitists and generalists began to evolve. If the doctor-nurse relationship reflected, as suggested by Oakley (1984), the family male dominance-female subservience relationship of husband and wife, then the relationship between a superintendent and her nurses could also be seen to reflect the mistress-servant relationship of the typical Victorian middle-class household.

To take the analogy further, servants were 'trained' not 'educated'. The education of nurses, along with the concept of State registration were not seen to be matters of prime concern in the early years. A modern historian comments of Florence Nightingale that 'she preferred patronage and surveillance of nurses lives to guiding their professional work' (Smith, 1982). She feared above all 'stereotyped mediocrity', and was afraid that registration, with its inevitable requirement of a uniform standard and examinations, would bring this about.

She appears to have had deep reservations concerning book learning related to nursing . . . 'unless it bear fruit it is all gilding and veneer' (Nightingale, 1888). The consequences arising from the way in which nurse training evolved, and the utilisation of an apprenticeship system meant an emphasis on 'doing' at the expense of 'knowing', and as time passed the development of an anti-academic bias, that was to exert a powerful and sometimes obstructive influence on the growth of nursing as a profession.

Very aptly did Carter comment in 1939 of this earlier period:

> Habits of discipline, unquestioning obedience, the lack of any criticism from the outside world, even from fellow workers, must have led to an acceptance of conditions which might have been improved had they been criticised.

Unfortunately nurses were trained to conform and accept, not criticise or question, as the foregoing account has demonstrated.

It has been suggested that when Nightingale

> conceived of the idea of training women to be nurses she envisaged such a training to be a socially accepted alternative to marriage for women who wanted that option, or as an acceptable occupation for married women . . . who fell on hard times.
>
> (Crowder, 1985)

As was noted earlier, there were few occupations open to women at the time, though the feminist movement was gathering strength towards the close of the nineteenth century, and coupled with the work of early women pioneers, some professions were beginning, albeit reluctantly, to accept small numbers of women into their ranks.

Nightingale was not herself an enthusiastic supporter of the feminist movement (though some of her writings, her refusal to accept for herself the traditional Victorian role for a woman of her social position, and her active and productive life suggest a degree of feminist thinking) and the movement itself did not turn its attention to nursing until the turn of the century.

Feminism has been defined as 'a world view that values women, and that confronts systematic injustices based on gender'. (Chinn and Wheeler, 1985). There are four major philosophical approaches to feminist theory. These are first, liberal feminism, which seeks to change the social, political and economic influences which contribute to lack of female power in society; secondly, Marxist philosophy which views women as exploited and oppressed both in domestic and industrial settings within a male-dominated, class-bound capitalist system; thirdly, socialist feminism, which looks beyond the Marxist approach to other cultural aspects of institutionalised gender discrimination, particularly related to the female role within the family; and, lastly, radical feminism which suggests that oppression of women exists within *all* economic systems, and requires not a change in economic, social or political systems to address the problems, but rather the development of women-centred systems. Women's experiences need to be analysed and valued, it is suggested, without the imposition of male ideology. Milauskas (1985) suggests '. . . female nurses are twice socialised – into subservience and traditionalism. First as women and second as workers in a work setting that mimics social roles'. Chapter 3 will explore this aspect further.

Though many would disagree strongly with the above position, it is of interest to address the basic tenet of feminism, that women constitute an oppressed group, and consider the group traits in relation to nursing as it has developed through the late nineteenth and early twentieth centuries. These traits include lack of self-esteem, lack of pride in nursing accompanied by failure to support or participate in professional organisations; and the demonstration of displaced aggression (horizontal violence) towards colleagues, often displayed both at the micro and macro levels of nursing activities; in addition to lack of autonomy, and control by others. Leaders in such groups have also been noted as having negative attributes; they are controlling, coercive and rigid (Roberts, 1983). Chapter 2 will explore these, and other psychological aspects related to group behaviour in greater depth.

These problems were not assisted, in terms of a more positive development, by a training experience which Sheahan, writing of schools of nursing, described as 'places where . . . women learned to be girls' (Sheahan, 1981).

Chapter 4 will explore in detail this aspect of nursing experience. The clinical context in which many nurses gained their practical experience tended to perpetuate the problem in being 'oppressive, reductionistic milieu of the patriarchal order – the hospital – which does not foster, endorse, nor approve nursing practice based on nursing's own theorics and valucs'. (Chinn and Wheeler, 1985). Although these are comments pertaining to the years of the mid twentieth century, the problems identified were extant from the earliest days. Chapter 7 will assess the problems in this area, examining both past and current experiences.

By the first decade of the twentieth-century nursing as an occupation (not yet a profession, though often accorded the courtesy title) was emerging as a socially heterogeneous, predominantly female grouping, subjected to strict discipline, operating within a hierarchical bureaucratic framework, poorly remunerated, and experiencing a continued relationship of dominance by, and subservience to the medical profession. Lovell (1981) comments that 'Dominant groups usually define the acceptable roles for the subordinate. These roles typically provide services that no dominant group member wants to perform.'

The dominant influence of the medical profession over nursing and nurse education was set to continue for a further half century; the handmaiden image was to die only very slowly. The so-called 'autonomy' of Nightingale nurses was less that of 'professional' individuals than that of a 'nursing structure', where the Matron was undisputed head of an independent department (Bellaby and Oribabor, 1980). The role of the nurse continued to be, and currently is still influenced by sexual role stereotyping.

Throughout the twentieth-century nursing has been endeavouring to move towards professional status. Intimately connected with this has been the protracted struggle for registration, attempts to improve training programmes, the introduction of degree courses, and repeated attempts to improve remuneration. All ultimately seeking thereby to raise standards of nursing care. Later chapters in this book will address these educational, political and ethical issues in depth.

There have, throughout the period however, been influences at work within nursing highly resistant to change, and seeking to preserve and perpetuate some aspects of nursing tradition no longer appropriate in the last decade of the twentieth century. These influences have often operated at a subtle level, providing what became known as the 'hidden agenda' within nurse education. Attitudes and values, hierarchical relationships, and philosophies of care are frequently transmitted as an integral part of student socialisation, and pressure to conform (sometimes with disastrous consequences) then exerted.

This book seeks, in the chapters that follow, to address these problems from a variety of perspectives, while this chapter has sought to indicate where the roots of some of the difficulties may have had their origins. The reader is brought round again to the quotation with which this chapter opened, and could perhaps usefully close with a warning from Nightingale herself that 'In seeking to prevent disasters in the future, it is wise to be guided by as many as possible of the lessons of the past' (1858).

References

Baly, M. (1986). Shattering the Nightingale myth. *Nursing Times and Nursing Mirror*, **82(24)**, 16–18.

Bedford Fenwick, E. (1888). The development of the art of nursing. *Nursing Record*, **1(29)**, 395–8.

Bellaby, P. and Oribabor, P. (1980). 'The history of the present' – contradiction and struggle in nursing. *In Rewriting Nursing History*, C. Davies (ed.), pp. 147–74. Croom Helm, London.

Boyd, N. (1982). *Josephine Butler, Octavia Hill, Florence Nightingale: Three Victorian Women who Changed their World*. Macmillan, London.

Branca, P. (1975). *Silent Sisterhood: Middle-class Women in the Victorian Home*. Croom Helm, London.

Briggs, A. (1983). *A Social History of England*. Weidenfeld & Nicolson, London.

Bullough, V. and Bullough, B. (1979). *The Care of the Sick: the Emergence of Modern Nursing*. Croom Helm, London.

Carter, G.B. (1939). *A New Deal for Nurses*. Gollancz, London.

Chinn, P.L. and Wheeler, C.E. (1985). Feminism and nursing. Can nursing afford to remain aloof from the women's movement? *Nursing Outlook*, **33(2)**, 74–7.

Crow, D. (1971). *The Victorian Woman*. Allen & Unwin, London.

Crowder, E.L.M. (1985). Historical perspectives of nursing's professionalism. *Occupational Health Nursing*, **33(4)**, 184–90.

Dannatt, A. (1888). What constitutes an efficient nurse. *Nursing Record*, **1(8)**, 87–90.

Davies, C. (1977). Continuities in the development of hospital nursing in Britain. *Journal of Advanced Nursing*, **2(5)**, 479–93.

Delamont, S. and Duffin, L. (eds) (1978). *The Nineteenth-century Woman: her Cultural and Physical World*. Croom Helm, London.

Garrett, E. (1867). Volunteer hospital nursing. *Macmillan's Magazine*, **15**, 494–9.

Lewis, J. (1984). *Women in England 1870–1950: Sexual Divisions and Social Change*. Wheatsheaf, Brighton.

Lovell, M.C. (1981). Silent but perfect 'partners': medicine's use and abuse of women. *Advances in Nursing Science*, **3(2)**, 25–40.

Manton, J. (1965). *Elizabeth Garrett Anderson*. Methuen, London.

Milauskas, J. (1985). Will nursing assert itself? *Nursing Administration Quarterly*, **9(3)**, 1–15.

Mollett, M. (1888). Discipline. *Nursing Record*, **1(9)**, 99–101.

Nightingale, F. (1858). *Subsidiary Notes as to the Introduction of Female Nursing into Military Hospitals in Peace and in War*. Harrison, London.

Nightingale, F. (1888). *To the Probationer Nurses in the Nightingale Fund School, at St Thomas's Hospital*. (Unpublished).

Nightingale, F. (1979). *Cassandra: an Essay*. Feminist Press, New York.

Oakley, A. (1984). What price professionalism? The importance of being a nurse. *Nursing Times*, **80(50)**, 24–7.

Palmer, I.S. (1983). Nightingale revisited. *Nursing Outlook*, **31(4)**, 229–33.

Prince, J. (1984). *Miss Nightingale's Vision of a Nursing Profession: an Interim Report*. Royal College of Nursing, London.

Rathbone, W. (1890). *Sketch of the History and Progress of District Nursing from its Commencement in the Year 1859 to the Present Date*. Macmillan, London.

Roberts, S.J. (1983). Oppressed group behavior: implications for nursing. *Advances in Nursing Science*, **5(4)**, 21–30.

Rundle, R.N. (1973). *Britain's Economic and Social Development from 1700 to the Present Day*. University of London Press, London.

Seymer, L. (1960). *Florence Nightingale's Nurses: the Nightingale Training School 1860–1960*. Pitman, London.

Sheahan, D. (1981). *Influence of Occupational Sponsorship on the Professional Development of Nursing*. Rockefeller Archives, Tarrytown, NY.

Smiles, S. (1859), *Self-help*. J Murray, London.

Smith, F.B. (1982). *Florence Nightingale: Reputation and Power*. Croom Helm, London.

Southgate, G. (1965). *English Economic History*. Dent, London.

Tennyson, A. (1953). *Poetical Works*. Oxford University Press, Oxford.

Thrift, N. and Williams, P. (eds) (1987). *Class and Space: the Making of Urban Society*. Routledge and Kegan Paul, London.

Trevelyan, G.M. (1946). *English Social History*, 2nd edn. Longman, London.

Vicinus, M. (ed.) (1972). *Suffer and Be Still: Women in the Victorian Age*. Indiana University Press, Bloomington, Ind.

Wheeler, C.E. (1985). The American Journal of Nursing and the socialization of a profession, 1900–1920. *Advances in Nursing Science*, **7(2)**, 20–34.

Whittaker, E. and Oleson, V. (1964). The faces of Florence Nightingale:

functions of the heroine legend in an occupational sub-culture. *Human Organization*, **23(2)**, 123–30.

Woodham-Smith, C. (1950). *Florence Nightingale 1820–1910*. Constable, London.

Woolf, V. (1929). *A Room of One's Own*. Hogarth, London.

2 The psychology of attitudes and values

Introduction

To take but a cursory glance at the historical perspectives of nursing one has to be impressed by the power of the transmission of values, attitudes and beliefs passed on so religiously from one generation to another. These social and psychological structures, which will be explored within this chapter, contribute to the art and science of nursing. They impact upon the delivery of care to the client and influence the relationships nurses have with each other and the multidisciplinary care team. It is only recently that critical scrutiny of what nursing is has generated the impetus to consider what part the transmission of values, attitudes and beliefs may play in either conforming to or challenging practice in nursing.

Within this chapter it is intended to review the current perspectives on attitudes and values, their purpose and their contribution to nursing. A generalist approach will be taken to encourage individuals exploring these ideas to reflect upon their own experiences of nursing, their socialisation into the profession and the part they play in the transmission of attitudes, values and beliefs within their professional practice.

The study of attitudes has been fueled by the belief that there is a strong relationship between attitudes and behaviour. If such a linear relationship exists, thought the social psychologists, it may be possible to gain insight, if not predict, the individual's behaviour. Allport (1954) viewed attitudes as 'the most distinctive and indispensable concept in social psychology'. Psychologists are also interested because the implication is that one can influence behavioural changes by changing attitudes.

The literature reveals numerous definitions of what attitudes are, each reflecting the belief system of the authors. Consequently psychologists are unlikely to agree upon any one definition. I wish to take a brief look at the various perspectives rather than to deliberate over the many definitions which readers may find in the literature. Hopefully from this exploration readers will be able to decide for themselves where they, or the author stands.

Attitudes – a structural approach

Secord and Backman (1964) propose that most definitions are comprised of three components:

1. The cognitive component, what the person thinks about a certain subject.
2. The affective component, what the person feels about a certain subject.
3. The behavioural component, how the person behaves towards a certain subject in the light of the individual's thoughts and feelings.

The simplicity of the view is rather naive as it is well known that human nature is less reliable or predictable due to the many individual and situational factors involved. One of the most reported studies is that by La Piere (1934). Travelling with a Chinese couple through the United States of America, he monitored the expression of cultural attitudes and prejudices that the couple experienced in attempting to obtain accommodation. La Piere writes that in 10,000 miles of travel discrimination was encountered once and there was no observation of prejudice. Following the travel, letters were then sent to the establishments which had been visited asking for their response to a request to provide accommodation and food to members of the Chinese culture. Results reveal a different picture from the actual experiences. Over 90% replied they would not offer hospitality, one replied they would offer hospitality and the remainder replied that they would have to take circumstances at the time into account. Presumably the circumstances being referred to are the personal judgements being made about the individuals in front of them and the circumstances at the time. Therefore perhaps all that can be proposed is that attitudes may demonstrate a predisposition towards a certain subject.

Discrepancy between what someone says and does would suggest that the study of attitudes is more complex and needs to take into account situational factors and the purpose that the attitude fulfils for the individual.

Fishbein and Ajzen (1975) suggest that beliefs, values and intentions need to be brought into the equation of attitude study thus enabling a much greater degree of specificity to be achieved (see Fig. 2.1). Beliefs represent the knowledge an individual holds about their world around them. Allport (1935) defines a value as 'a belief upon which a man acts by preference'. It refers then to a quality or property of a thing that makes it useful, desired or esteemed. It is not the value of the thing that is of importance but the role the thing has (Reber, 1985). Values may be also held by a society or a profession whereby cultural, social or professional norms are held and transmitted; for example the United Kingdom Central Council for Nursing (UKCC) Professional Code of Conduct for Nurses (1984).

Newcomb (1950) suggests that an attitude may be defined as a 'learned predisposition to respond in a consistently favourable or unfavourable manner with respect to a given object'. Pennington (1986) suggests that this definition incorporates four important aspects of attitudes relating to the structural approach:

1. Attitudes are learned through experience.
2. Attitudes predispose people to respond in a certain way.
3. Attitudes predispose the person to be consistent in their response.
4. Attitudes are evaluated by the holder.

In the light of his proposal Pennington offers a structural analysis of how these statements may be diagrammatically represented (see Fig. 2.2).

A critical view of his proposal would be that he has not elaborated upon his first statement, that attitudes are learned through experience. It is essential to consider all forms of learning, not only a cognitive perspective of structured information processing, but also the power of social learning (Bandura, 1977A) whereby vicarious learning, that is learning through observation, provides the richest source of information from which to process complex life experiences from our social world.

Although within the literature most studies of attitudes refer to the individual as the holder of the attitude I would propose that it is also the social experience, (particularly within nursing as this is what we are concerned with in this chapter) which is the holder of attitudes, and powerful in the sharing and transmission of the attitudes of a profession. Thus attitudes may be held by a reference group which become accessible to others by gaining membership of that reference group.

Pennington (1986) includes values as a contributory influence to attitudes (see Fig. 2.2). Values are standards that guide behaviour. Kilmann (1981) suggests that 'they are guides to what needs, wants, and desires people should have, what interests, preferences and goals are seen as desirable or undesirable, what individual dispositions or traits one ought to have, and what beliefs and attitudes individuals should expres'. Kilmann also states that a knowledge of values should explain and predict a persons behaviour as values underlie differences in beliefs, attitudes and behaviour (Rokeach, 1973: Sedhom, 1982). Feldman and Newcomb (1969) develop this further suggesting that each individual can reflect a unique combination of values in the aspects of theoretical, economic, aesthetic, social, political and religious values. This view brings one closer to the recognition of the complexities of value systems held. Values may not appear to be congruent to the observer, but are constructed as so by the individual in order for their unique relationship to their world to be sustained.

Values are determined by cultural and societal influences and also occupational groups. Allport, et al. (1970) found that different occupational groups revealed distinctive value profiles and O'Neill (1975) suggests that choice of

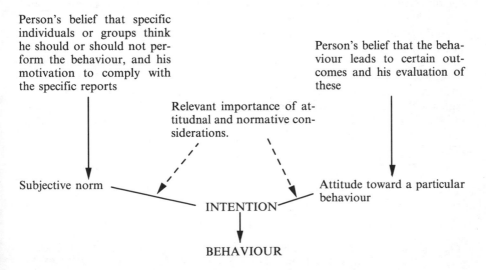

Fig. 2.1   Ajzen and Fishbein's (1980) Theory of reasoned action

occupation is related to the values a person possesses, aspires to, or associates with the occupation. Homans in 1950 described the importance of a shared value system to group and organizational life suggesting that the commitment to the value system is necessary for the groups survival and to the effectiveness of the group's work (cited by Homans, 1961). Values therefore influence not only the attitudes an individual holds but perhaps also the choice of career aspired to.

An additional structural perspective of attitudes is contained in the view that we have developed, through our experience, a schema of attitudes. The concept of a schema arises from the cognitive school within social psychology. The schema is a cognitive structure which guides the processing of and retrieval of information. It may be likened to a filing system, whereby all the information processed is stored in a logical and related way, and relationships can be seen to exist between the various files held in the filing cabinet. A similar view is held in relation to us holding a schema for person perception, which from the literature is known to be fraught with bias and inaccuracy. The attitude schema can also be viewed as possibly providing the individual with a somewhat narrow and biased perspective, due to our tendency to pay most attention to information from our environment which is relevant to currently held attitudes, thus lifting or inhibiting recognition of attitude relevant information that may be neutral, irrelevant or challenging. A common accusation is that of being 'narrow minded'; perhaps such a statement reveals the inherent difficulties of utilising schemas to process information. However, by being aware of the potential limitations the schema may set us, recognition of this may permit us to traverse this psychological boundary.

Fiske and Linville (1980) say that the research into schema concepts is as yet limited and worthy of more attention, especially as the schema is evidently dynamic, responsive to experience, may not be static, and is culturally and socially grounded. The schema may provide a versatile method of storing and understanding complex knowledge.

Additionally this view permits the dynamic and persistent search for new understanding, new meaning or acquiring new perspectives which individuals may engage in. This may be of significance when considering the formation of attitudes. In terms of information-processing Craik and Lockhart (1972 cited by Gross, 1990) proposed the idea that perhaps complements the rather rigid mechanistic model described by notable researchers such as Ebbinghaus (1885, cited by Hebb, 1949), Broadbent (1958) and Atkinson and Shiffrin

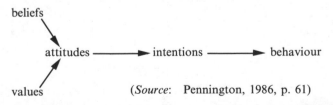

(*Source*: Pennington, 1986, p. 61)

Fig. 2.2 Structural analysis of attitudes showing the relationships between beliefs, values, intentions and behaviour. Reproduced from Pennington (1986) with permission

(1977). Craik and Lockhart suggest that it is the nature of the stimulus and the time available to the individual which determines the 'level' of processing that takes place; recognising therefore that the human being is perhaps not as thorough in the processing of information as some researchers may like to think. There are three levels of processing;

1. Structural or shallow level.
2. Phonetic or phonemic level.
3. Semantic level.

The first level is considered to be superficial, and the following two of increasing depth; suggesting that at the deeper level more meaningful analysis is taking place and therefore it is more likely that the events will be recalled. It is not the encoding of the stimuli into the memory that is of significance, but rather that at the deeper levels of processing there is greater elaboration of memories thus facilitating association between new material and existing memories (Festinger and Carlsmith, 1959). Perhaps attitude formation and development is also dependent upon the depth of processing. As we will see later the socialisation experience is often overwhelming and rapid, prohibiting the opportunity for depth analysis of exposure to attitudes, and hence a rapid adoption of the expressed attitudes, values and beliefs. For example it is, perhaps, easier for students to be seen to adopt behaviours observed in nurses in the practice setting than to challenge, and be seen not to comply with the work ethic by questioning (Melia, 1987).

There are a number of theories referring to the development of attitudes that operate with a schema foundation. They are described as the family of Consistency Theories. Heider (1958) for example proposed a Balance Theory in which he said that people seek to find harmony amongst their attitudes, values, and beliefs; thus consistency would be found within an individual's views and statements about life. Contributing to this harmonious state are our judgements of attitudes held by others in that we utilise our attitude schema to make judgements whilst searching for understanding about the attitudes operating within the social group. Such a harmonious view was challenged by Festinger (1957) and Festinger and Carlsmith (1959) who recognised that an individual could hold two cognitions simultaneously which were psychologically inconsistent. (Take a few minutes to reflect upon your own experiences; can you recall holding two cognitions which are inconsistent with one another? One example may be when working in a clinical environment where nursing care is based upon a primary nursing philosophy which is held to be good, yet there also exists an unwritten rule of tasks having to be done by a certain grade of nurse personnel.) The theory is known as Dissonance Theory, and cognitive dissonance can be extremely uncomfortable.

What then happens to the inconsistent attitudes? Osgood and Tannen-baum's Congruity Theory (1955) maintains that the attitude which is held less firmly will change in order for the individual to attain congruity and diminish cognitive dissonance. Before briefly looking at what factors may influence attitude change let us consider the second major perspective upon atttitudes; that is, what function do attitudes serve for the individual?

Attitudes – A Functional Approach

Four specific functions are proposed (McGuire, 1969; Katz 1960). These are the *adaptive* function which contributes to the individual achieving their desires. This may manifest itself in the individual adopting certain attitudes similar to those held by others who currently are achieving what the individual desires. This may mean role modelling behaviour, or identification with a role model. The *knowledge* function of attitudes concerns the information the person holds about the environment they are in, enabling the world to appear a little more familiar and even predictable.

Stereotyping is a popular strategy employed to do this, but it possesses the limitations of oversimplification of the environmental stimuli and also the risk of making assumptions. Attempts to make the world predictable is an unprofitable strategy to employ in order to maintain one's attitudes.

The *self-expressive* function lies close to the ideas of self-perception theory. Bem (1967) describes how attitudes may develop from observation of our own behaviour. The understanding we have of ourselves comes from analysis of ours and others interactions with ourselves in a range of environments over time. Some self-perceptions may be held over a very long period of time and may be resistent to change in spite of much disconfirmation. Erikson's work (1967 cited by Erikson, 1968) on psychosocial crises will provide further reading to develop this psychoanalytic perspective. Some attitudes however may be easily influenced if facilitating the meeting of a need or contributing to the ego defensive function. This function is to protect the self-image, particularly from others, that the individual holds of themselves. Essentially the attitudes one holds about oneself are balanced by both positive and negative attributes and may be a measure of our self-esteem.

This functional approach identifies the two prerequisites for influencing attitude change, or the successful transmission of attitudes; namely what the person's attitude is and secondly the purpose the attitude, or the new attitude, serves for the individual.

Now let us briefly consider the key elements in influencing attitude change.

Factors influencing attitude change

The key components of persuasive communication are the source, the message, the recipient and the situation in which the communication is taking place. Each of the components has key factors to be considered.

The status of the sender of the message has a very powerful effect upon the receiver's impression of the message. If the source is seen as credible and has status and authority then it is more likely that the attitude will be influenced. If the intentions of the sender of the information are considered trustworthy then this also contributes to the effectiveness of the attitude transmission. Within nursing's historical image, there is a belief in the altruistic or spiritual aspect of the calling that permeates through the lay population. This may therefore strongly colour the student nurse's belief about the trustworthiness of the sender of the message. In other words whatever the ward sister or charge nurse says 'must' be right, certainly in the patient's best interest, or in the student's best interest. This process contributes to the very commonly cited 'theory-practice gap'. Often the attitudes and practice perceived during clinical practice experience are adopted rather than that of the research-based education discussed within the college environment. The student is sensitive to the cognitive dissonance (Festinger, 1957) being experienced and this is managed by the student by responding to the most powerful stimulus at the time. Through observation of the clinical staff the student identifies with the practices and behaviours which are rewarded, or given feedback to, the social group on the ward. Within the college setting the student aspires to the curriculum set by the educator.

Motivation to be a part of the ward team is very powerful. Therefore the need to maintain cognitive consistency is strong. The student will therefore modify his or her behaviour in order to demonstrate the adoption of the ward's collective attitudes, or the college collective attitudes, depending upon the situational demands.

The attractiveness of the sender refers to how the person is seen by the receiver of the message. The role model of senior nurses within a nursing hierarchy hold all the credentials equipping them to be extremely effective sources of attitude change.

The effectiveness of the receiver's response to the actual message would seem to be most influenced by the significance of the message for that receiver. If the adoption of an attitude facilitates the socialisation passage into the nursing culture the motivation is very powerful for the individual or the group of new recruits.

The function that attitudes fulfil for the individual is elaborated in the work of Katz (1960) already mentioned, as we shall see when discussing the process of the transmission of attitudes. Within the process of learning nursing the adaptive function of attitudes is of paramount importance. To be accepted by nurses seen as 'already successful' and part of the professional culture, it is almost worth foregoing all the attitudes previously held and adopting the attitudes of the new culture and society.

The student then is exposed to both an explicit curriculum of education and also a hidden curriculum (See Chapter 4). Snyder (1971) defines the hidden curriculum as 'the implicit demands (as opposed to the explicit obligations of the visible curriculum) that are found in every learning institution and which students have to find out and respond to in order to survive within it, thus the central task of the hidden curriculum for the student is to learn which patterns of behaviour are tribally and/or institutionally sanctioned'.

The credibility and status of the sender of the message, 'nurses in the know' are powerful in both position and as potential sanctioner to join or stay within the profession.

Social learning theory – the contribution to attitude transmission

Social learning theory is proposed by members of the behavioural school of psychology in an attempt to further develop ideas away from the traditionalist views, such as Pavlov (1927), Watson (1928) and Skinner (1938), cited by Atkinson et al. 1990 of behaviour occurring as a consequence of reinforcement the individual received following a particular behaviour. They were more interested in emphasising the interaction between the individual and the environment and they additionally recognised the presence of the cognitive processes within the individual experience. Bandura (1977a) emphasises that a major tenet of social learning theory is that of vicarious learning, or learning through observation.

Observation of the behaviour of others is possibly the most profitable strategy afforded to the individual, as learning the skills of interpersonal interaction would otherwise be extremely labour – intensive and no doubt fraught with difficulty if we were only able to acquire the skills through strict behavioural convention. In fact social learning theory is the major route from which these skills are acquired; observing how others act in a social situation and noting the consequences of the interaction. This strategy of learning often takes place with no specific intention on the observer's part or on the part of the model (the person being observed) or with the observer receiving a specific reinforcement. The reward of remembering how a person behaved in a specific situation, and what the consequences were is sufficient in itself. However, it is the consequences that influence whether or not the observed behaviours will be integrated and used in the individual's repertoire of behaviours (Bandura et al., 1961). One of the significant variables affecting the likelihood of imitation is thought to be the characteristics of the model observed.

The registered nurse and student nurse (models) may be of sufficient status to fulfil the newcomer's (observer) 'ideal' role model. Observation of these people will be essential to enable initial forays into the care environment.

One factor of importance is the idea of *latent learning*. Observed behaviour does not need to reveal itself in the immediate future, but may be revealed much later when the interaction of the individual and the environment is appropriate. Hence initial experiences of observing a caring interaction may be initiated by the observer later in their nursing experience.

An additional element of social learning theory is the significance of *self-regulatory processes*. This is the individual setting standards for themselves in terms of acceptability, of appropriateness; and also highlights the cognitive processing by the individual that contributes to the performing of behaviour.

Standards may be set by a professional organisation, as in the United Kingdom Central Council (UKCC) Code Of Professional Conduct (1984), against which the individual will judge the observed behaviour.

Attribution theory – explaining the behaviour of others

When observing others we are engaging in a deliberate process of trying to understand why a person behaved in a certain way. What were their motives or their intentions? It is suggested that this activity enables us, through our perception, to then make sense of our own world more effectively.

This question was initially asked by Heider (1958), the founding father of attribution theory. Heider suggested that we attempt to understand behaviour by attributing causality to either an internal or an external cause; these are the two main kinds of attribution.

An internal or personal attribution means that the individual is seen as responsible, or to blame, for the performed behaviour. An internal attribution always seems to carry the implication of intention to act.

An external or situational attribution means that the behaviour observed is seen as a consequence of the environment, situationally determined, and therefore no one is seen as responsible.

It has been suggested by Nisbett and Ross (1980) that there is a risk of over-emphasising personal responsibility when making attributions; they have coined the term *fundamental attribution error*. The reason for this remains somewhat unclear. However it may be because of our need to make sense of the world as the environment is a constantly changing place and often impossible to control. Therefore if we place responsibility for behaviour on an individual then perhaps it enables us to feel more confident and safe in a complex world.

This leads to one of the criticisms of attribution theory; that it provides no context or frame of reference indicating the past experiences of the individual, or the historical and cultural understanding and interpretations of behaviour that are learnt through the socialisation process. Attribution theory risks viewing individuals sense making as too clinical as opposed to part of a rich tapestry of making sense of the world.

Kelley (1967) developed his work from Heider by focusing his studies upon the judgements of internal and external causality. He attempted to provide the understanding for explaining behaviour. His Model of Co-variation is only usable when the observer has exposure to the person over a period of time. The principle of co-variation is the analysis of the behaviour observed over time. Kelley suggests three types of information are used to estimate attribution of a particular behaviour.

1. *Distinctiveness*: the extent to which the person normally behaves in this way.
2. *Consistency*: the extent to which the person has behaved in this way previously.
3. *Consensuality*: the extent to which other people behave in a similar way.

Kelley's model may be one tool in understanding how the student, new to a situation, may attempt to understand nurses behaviour and then their consequent attitudes which are seen to contribute to the behaviour performed.

The tendency to make internal attribution was further explored by Jones and Davis (1965) who suggested that the goal of attribution is to be able to infer that both the behaviour and intention to produce the behaviour corresponds to an underlying disposition, or stable personal quality, of the person observed. In order to understand what information contributed to making these correspondent inferences they propose four sources:

1. That the behaviour is seen as socially desirable; that it represents the norms or the socially sanctioned behaviour within the situation observed.

2. That the behaviour is part of the person's role; the behaviour being role driven rather than person driven.
3. Prior expectations of the person being observed. If the observer familiar with the person, prior knowledge may contribute to the process of inference. Especially if the observed behaviour confirms previous attributions made about underlying dispositions.
4. The fourth factor is that of free will; is the behaviour seen as an act of choice or is it situationally determined?

Nisbett and Ross (1980) comment on two further errors or bias which may affect attribution, that of *actor or observer error*. Here individuals or groups of people view their performed behaviour as a result of the situational influences, as opposed to it being personal responsibility; yet perceive the behaviour of *others* as being of personal responsibility.

The third type of error, the *false consensus effect* is the tendency an individual has to assume that other peoples' behaviour is likely to be more similar to their own than it really is.

One can see that the many variables and factors influencing the attribution process makes one question any judgement that may be reached! So why then do we engage in the process in the first place? Hewstone (1983) suggests three major reasons:

1. The need to promote self-esteem, to acknowledge success, and to manage failure which must be due to an external cause.
2. To be able to effectively portray oneself to others in terms of self-presentation.
3. To be able to establish some sense of control over the social world through explanation and prediction.

There may also be, then, a self-serving bias in our attributional endeavours.

In addition to these theories one must take into account the socialisation experiences through which others, more familiar with the new social world enable the newcomer in their sense-making by interpreting the behaviour of others (Berger and Luckman, 1966) or through prior warning of how to behave. Readers may recall the numerous conversations taking place in the sluice about how to behave in difficult circumstances, or what behaviour is acceptable or unacceptable in a forthcoming clinical experience. Therefore the transmission of attitudes, values and beliefs has occurred; being components of the survival package in that they are crucial aspects to the sense-making, and the information processing, of the perceived social behaviour.

Social cognition

Theories of social cognition recognise the dynamic interaction between the individual and the environment. It is not a straightforward process in understanding why people behave or not in certain ways in certain circumstances, Human nature is consistently intriguing. These theories include the attribution theories, decision-making theories and schema theories – all attempting to understand how individuals makes sense of the world around them. Perhaps what is important to recognise is that the complexities involved in the 'making sense' inevitably are influenced by the individual's cultural, historical and personal uniqueness, and that what is of particular importance is the enabling of the individual in understanding the whys and wherefores of their actions representing their attitudes, values and beliefs. To facilitate becoming a knowledgeable practitioner as opposed to employing tacit knowledge takes into account the dialectical paradigm of psychology (Buss, 1979).

Dialectical theorists are particularly interested in the interface between the individual's image, understanding of, and reality of the world with the world that is constructed for the individual through social and cultural forces. The ideas are not so much to seek an understanding of the individual's explanation of the world, as to understand the social, cultural, and historical forces that influence making sense of the world. Into this equation would come the social, cultural, historical and experiential forces that influenced the individual to choose nursing as an occupation, as well as his or her uniqueness in responding to experience. Further, how do these then contribute to the individual's experience and development of their delivery of professional nursing care? This is a question for future study.

Socialisation – its contribution to the teaching of attitudes values and beliefs

The individual student enters through the portals of the chosen hospital excited and eager in anticipation about the future career they are about to commence. Often a sense of 'having arrived' accompanies the sense of just starting a major transition phase. Many of you reading this chapter may choose to reflect for a moment or two upon your memories of those first experiences of arriving.

Merton (1957) describes the preparatory expectations as 'anticipatory socialisation', a rich and sophisticated personal understanding of the role, nature and purpose of the nurse. There are numerous variables contributing to this understanding, including observation of the professionals, media information, personal experience of health care, vicarious experiences and other members of the individual's social system, who readily contribute to the understanding of their potential future role (see Chapter 3).

Thus, with the person comes a range of individual and societal expectations about the role of the nurse and how this person ideally sees themselves becoming a nurse. The investment is very important in that it is tied inextricably to the person's concept of self. Burns (1980) defines self concept as 'the set of attitudes a person holds towards himself'. The self-concept is composed of self-image, self-esteem and the ideal self (Gross, 1987) and is formed through developmental phases and life experiences. These experiences may be success, failure or humiliation, and their impact on the self-concept will also be affected by those people who were part of the experiences, namely significant others such as parents, peers, teachers or authority figures. All these contribute to how the individual perceives himself, how the person portrays him or herself to others, and inevitably plays a part in occupational choice. In sum, the initial phase of entry into a new occupation brings an individual whose concept of self ensures they are not only highly motivated to become a member of the nursing profession but also vulnerable to, and therefore may be eager to adopt, the profession's attitudes values and beliefs.

Within this first phase of socialisation is a process of 'homogenising' (Davis, 1990) or 'divestiture' (Glaser and Strauss, 1971). Usually greeted with an element of excitement, the wearing of a uniform and thus being seen as a legitimate member of the institution contributes to the feeling of being welcomed, to feel part of the institution and to enhance self-esteem. It is not seen as a subtle degradation (Bradby, 1990) but of 'having arrived'. No doubt though, the seeds of subservience are sown, resulting in the nurturing and transmission of pre-selected professional attitudes and behaviour patterns (see Chapters 1 and 3).

Conformity can now be assured! The student is psychologically dependent upon their need to belong. If one briefly considers Maslow's theory of motivation (1954), cited by Maslow (1987) the individual is anxious to fulfil their need to belong in order to maintain their esteem needs. Maslow proposed that the individual is required to sufficiently fill the invariant sequence of need level before being enabled to move upwards to finally achieve self actualisation. The hierarchy of human needs progresses from lower to higher needs in the following sequence: physiological needs, safety needs, love and belonging needs, esteem needs, and self-actualization needs. The level of sufficiency is determined by the individual, thus enabling their innate drive towards their ultimate higher achievement.

The need to belong is essential in order for students to be confident in their selection and commitment to their choice of career on arrival at the hospital. Dissonance theory (Aronson and Mills, 1959) shows that the more effort an individual puts into achieving a certain goal, the more attractive and worthwhile it is perceived to be when it is finally achieved. Dissonance theory is also saying that regardless of how attractive the goal is it is what the person goes through to achieve it that is important (Pennington, 1986). It is the amount of effort and the investment to achieve that motivates the individual to seek acceptance by the profession they are joining; hence a potential distinct avoidance of challenge to attitudes, values and beliefs expressed. Disagreement becomes impossible, it is as though they are in a catch-22 situation, wanting to belong but also wanting to challenge, with loss of self-esteem being the painful casualty. For the majority of new students the risk of not belonging is the deterrent ensuring the individual remains within the group and the apprenticeship system determines conformity to the norms of the occupational group.

Bradby (1990) describes, in her study of the socialisation of student nurses in 1983, how group affinity had little contribution to make to enhancing the individual's self-esteem except in adversity. She found that students maintained their self-perception by retaining links with social contacts outside the professional system.

Bem (1967) suggests that a person forms their attitudes through observation of themselves; self-perception theory. Initial contact with a new socialisation system may be a stressful experience, and as a consequence the individual seeks familiar social contact to maintain self-concept and self-esteem. Satisfaction of esteem needs is a potent motivator that depends upon both the opinion that others hold of the subject's position and the subject's own evaluation (Neidermeyer and Neidermeyer, 1986). The maintenance of social support may facilitate the transition process for the individual. Social support has been discussed in terms of it's buffering potential to stress by Cohen and Wills (1985) and by many other authors. It would seem to be a fruitful area of research to consider how social support systems mitigate against stress, distress and disease (Caplan, 1974; Cobb, 1976, Sarason and Sarason 1985). The term 'buffer' is used to indicate the protective enhancement it proffers for the person. Its relationship to the socialisation experience has not been explored, however, as an indicator of how an individual may behave, and its role in supporting self-esteem (Hilbert and Allen, 1985) whilst addressing new 'rites-de-passage' is of interest and worthy of future study.

Enquiring about the experiences of other students ahead in the apprenticeship system would reveal only confirmation that they too had been through the process, and 'look, they have survived'; thus contributing to both conformity and transmission of accepted codes of experiences and behaviour. Cohesiveness of thought, attitudes and behaviour may be seen as an effective method of dealing with emergencies and coping with anxiety (Menzies, 1970). The student exposed to such methods 'catches' this professional practice and prepares to teach others the code.

A norm is defined by the *Shorter Oxford Dictionary* (1973) as 'a rule or authoritative standard'. The standard is comprised of aims, beliefs and values developed by a group which relate particularly to the purposes of that group (Wilkins, 1976). There are expectations that members will behave according to the norms, establishing what then becomes 'normal' behaviour. Durkheim (1858–1917, cited by Wilkins, 1976) a French sociologist, suggests that the norms can only be internalised by individuals over a period of time. The length of time is not clear, except to say that exposure to the norms is a prerequisite. Some literature suggests a period of six to ten months (Louis, 1980; Bradby, 1990) yet perhaps for some, internalisation of the norms is never achieved. Might it be that these individuals recognise the society norms as constricting, and not complimentary to their own belief system. Some individuals have a strong enough self-esteem to enable non-conformity, while some may leave the institution. The apprenticeship system is powerful in enabling the student to 'learn the ropes' both in skills and attitudes, facilitated by a range of strategies, but particularly through role modelling.

Role modelling is one of the ways in which an individual builds and develops social roles. Dotan et al. (1986) found that role models are used by nurses through all the stages of professional life.

The role model is selected by the individual, often unbeknown to the role model him/herself. They are seen as 'an individual who possesses certain skills and displays techniques that the individual lacks and from whom, by observation and comparison with his own performance the individual can learn' (Kemper, 1968). The literature reveals a range of characteristics and qualities that may influence the choice of role model but Shuval and Adler (1980) suggest that it is not only the qualities of the role model but the values and norms that they represent which is important. Through observation the individual identifies complex interpersonal interaction and then gradually attempts to integrate these into their own repertoire. Inclusive within this process will be the behavioural features of attitudes, values and beliefs. Recognition of the power of role modelling has brought about the formalisation of this strategy in terms of preceptorship, mentorship and supervision of nurse learners.

Normative integration is one of the three different types of group integration described by Wilkins (1976). Mechanical integration refers to the group members becoming dependent upon one another as a result of division of labour. Found in the clinical area most evidently, but also in the college environment where more contemporary strategies for educational enterprise are employed, as opposed to the traditional 'chalk and talk'. Socio-psychological integration refers to the mutual satisfaction which takes place because of membership of the group. This may be seen to refer to the mutuality of team work engaged in relating to the care of clients. Normative integration refers to group members being held together by consensus of opinion and attitude. It is through this consistency of norms that support and a sense of belonging are reaffirmed. Wilkins writes that even if some individuals may have difficulty in compromising, inconsistency being minimally tolerated, the advantages of being a member outweigh the disadvantages of being outside. Hence commitment to attitudes and values are an inherent component of survival within the chosen group. Non-commitment may be met by ostracism or sanction.

Additionally, the individual is saturated with new stimuli which require situation or cultural-specific interpretation schemas in order to respond with meaningful and appropriate actions. Generally this is impossible and the individual is guided by role models and other team members. Thus individuals are behaving in congruence with the profession's attitudes, values and beliefs. Any inconsistency acts as an irritant or stimulus that motivates the individual to modify or change their attitudes to facilitate coherence or cognitive consistency (Atkinson et al. (1990).

Tedeschi et al. (1971) describe this as 'impression management' where the person is concerned with maintaining a consistency between their beliefs and their portrayal of attitudes to others. Time, opportunity and permission are essential prerequisites to reflection which is essential in order to enable self-generated attitude change.

Educational influence

In 1957 Merton described the phenomena of professional socialisation as an educational process whereby the individual, aspiring to become a member of a particular occupational group, develops a self-image which reflects the values and beliefs of that group. He goes further in describing occupational socialisation as 'the process by which proper selectively acquired values and attitudes, interests, skills and knowledge, in short, the culture current in the group to which they are or seek to become a member. It refers to the learning of social roles' (p. 248).

Initially, it is the educationalists in the college of nursing who are the role models aspired to by the student nurses. But until recently, the apprenticeship system of training and education has fostered a discrepancy between the theory and practice of nursing which has been blamed for the cavern between the educational curriculum and the curriculum of practice into which the taught attitudes have fallen, and within which the practice attitudes observed have flourished, the clinical staff being the cultivators.

Traditionally, education has been seen as unimportant, as caring (a feminine trait) is instinctive (Salvage, 1985). Fortunately, the traditional view, often founded on ritual and routine (see Chapter 1) is challenged essentially by professional moves to underpin practice with research-based knowledge, and most importantly, by the move of nursing education into higher educational forums.

This radical change, formalised by the UKCC in 1986 as Project 2000, enables the student of nursing studies to be a real student, not an apprentice. In fact the scene is set to promote the education of a practitioner of nursing who builds nursing practice and nursing knowledge upon a research base and upon reflective activities.

This move was precipitated by Argyris and Schon's (1974; 1978) work exploring the learning of expert professional nursing. It is the opportunity to reflect upon action that will influence both the understanding of that action and its consequences and of the variables that influence a particular action. For example, it may be realised that the reason for acting in a specific way may come from routines with a historical or sociological root (see Chapters 1 and 3). Only through opportunity to explore these variables will the individual be empowered to initiate self-generated change.

The process of self-monitoring (Bem, 1972) affords the individual opportunity to recognise situational cues and the responses of others before making decisions about their consequent behaviour (high self-monitors). This facilitates effective and creative problem-solving. Individuals who respond to their own internal experiences (low self-monitors) tend rarely to change their behaviour as a consequence of the social situation, staying true to the behavioural norms they have already established for themselves in terms of attitudes, values and beliefs. This may mean that the low self-monitor runs the risk of behaving according to custom and practice, ritual and routine.

Schon (1983) goes further to describe reflection-in-action whereby the practitioner recognises that the theory and action are inseparable and realises their use in action. Reflection-in-action enables active, flexible and creative problem-solving contributing to reflective conversation (Schon, 1983).

Schon emphasises that professional practice is individual to the practitioner enabling personalisation of action. Thus nursing knowledge moves from being tacit to acknowledged, understood and shared practice; bringing with it the potential for creativity in practice for the future.

This has particular importance for qualified nursing staff, recognised by the profession in its promotion of continuing educational opportunities of Post Registration Education and Practice Project, PREPP, (1990) and the English National Board Higher Award (1990), both of which seek to equip the practitioner for their increasing professional desire to harness theory to practice and to facilitate the next generation of students. Utilising the principles of reflective practice, a purposeful and goal directed activity (Boud et al. 1985), practitioners may enable the disempowering of ritual, routine and the attempts to maintain the status quo. Exposure to new perspectives inevitably encourages attitude change and an atmosphere of permissive questioning of values and norms in nursing care. Increasingly, nurses are engaged in higher education. This is essential as the profound change occurring within the profession has the potential for undermining the self-concept through questioning. So to engage in the challenge of questioning is more likely to be empowering than undermining when done collectively. The formal relationship of preceptorship may enhance this further (Dobbs, 1988).

This picture is in stark contrast to the previous image that 'the qualified nurses know but the students don't' to a mutual sharing. Hence the need to hold and promote fixed attitudes become less charged by fear and control.

The changing role of the nurse educator

With the change in nursing curricula allowing for provision of diploma studies in nursing, namely Project 2000, and degree studies, so too came the necessary review of the nurse educationalist role, and discussion and debate is set to continue concerning this matter. The opportunity to address the theory-practice gap which exists between the taught, and the caught attitudes, values and beliefs need not escape the professional. The essential requirement is for the college nurse educationalist to become familiar with the nurse practitioner in the practice setting in order to develop an educational enterprise which is both complementary, professional and for the benefit of the clients, the nurse learners and the patients.

The nurse-practitioner role manifests itself through many interpretations, indeed the lecturer-practitioner role combines facets of both roles. It is crucial for these subtleties to be both acknowledged and shared in terms of enhancing the professional experiences of teaching and learning.

Initial student experiences within Project 2000 involve a higher proportion of time spent within a college environment, the student being primarily exposed to the attitude, values and beliefs of the educationalist. Research studies within the graduate programme in America support the view that this professional socialisation (Crocker and Brodie, 1974; Conway, 1983), by the educationalists is due to the close proximity of faculty views. However, increasing the contact with the clinical practitioners may alter the attitudes, values and beliefs portrayed by the senior students, (Kramer and Schmalenberg, 1977) as the student experiences the dissonance or conflict between the taught and caught attitude, value and belief norm. Kramer (1974) referred to this experience as 'reality shock'; the finding that theoretical conceptions of the role of the nurse, and his or her role-relevant attitudes, values and beliefs, and the demands of the real work situation as being very different. Olsson and Gullberg (1988) propose that if variance exists between role congruence and role conception the potential for optimal attainment in professional knowledge and skills may be impeded.

Project 2000 students require educational opportunities that reflect reality-based, research-based professional practice; with articulated attitudes, values and beliefs which are shared by nurse educators, be they predominantly college or practice setting based.

The roles of the educator may be numerous depending upon the specific needs and requirements of the clinical situation and the nursing staff within the environment. The facilitation of qualified nurses as mentors (Puetz, 1985; Hagerty, 1986) or supervisors (Jones, 1982) may be essential for the educational role of the nurse to be facilitated. The aim, therefore is to enhance the theory, practice and self-efficacy (Bandura, 1977b; 1986) of qualified nurses in order that they may confidently challenge their own practice, whilst maintaining an effective self-concept, and thereby be empowered to facilitate the learning of the student nurse.

Self-efficacy is the belief that one has about one's own ability to successfully perform a specific behaviour; the behaviour being a desired one. Self-efficacy is important to consider when the learner commences the educational experiences equipping them to perform the much desired behaviours of a nurse. These are likely to be high when an individual enters a professional career of their choice (Lent and Hackett, 1987).

Self-efficacy expectations develop from four principal sources;

1. *From experience*, where repeated success increases self-efficacy.
2. *From vicarious learning*, where observation of others enables appraisal of self-efficacy. This is within the reference frame of role modelling.
3. *Through verbal persuasion by others*, in fact this source has the greatest effect on self-efficacy.
4. *From physiological information*, anxiety is a variable likely to diminish self-efficacy if there is too much, though a little acts as a motivator (de Vries *et al.*, 1988).

What is of significance is the contribution the individual's cognitive appraisal of the self-efficacy information makes to behaviour and their adoption of attitudinal behaviour. If an individual's self-efficacy is high then they may not be persuaded to behave according to situational norms or attitudes unless they perceive these to be congruent with their own professional view. However, if the situation should be determined by others and the individual perceives they have a low self-efficacy then they may behave according to the prescription of the situation.

Bandura (1977b) indicates that self-efficacy expectations vary along three dimensions;

1. *Magnitude*. this refers to the difficulty of the task.
2. *Generality*. which refers to whether the efficacy expectation can be generalized to other behaviours.
3. *Strength*. refering to the judgement of self-efficacy as to the individual's ability to perform the behaviour.

So, for example, challenging a senior nurse about prescribed care may be beyond the individual's judgement of their ability to act in both magnitude and in strength, even though in other situations they are well able to speak their mind, thus also indicating that the generality is low.

Self-efficacy is an essential variable to consider within the Fishbein and Ajzen (1980) model of behavioural intention (see Fig. 2.3). Additionally, self-efficacy needs recognition within the model proposed by Pennington (1986) (see Fig. 2.4).

The aim for the educator is thus to enable, through partnership with qualified and student nurses, maximum opportunity to attain quality, research-based, reflective practice. Minimising the use of tacit knowledge and the unauthorised power of attitudinal ritual in practice.

Conclusion

Attitudes, values and beliefs are integral and essential components of behaviour and may be indicators of a predisposition to act or 'make sense' of experiences in a particular way.

The socialisation process by which an individual comes to appreciate and know the attitudes, values and beliefs of the organisation they have sought to become a member of is a primary source of attitudes, values and beliefs being 'taught and caught'. In this way advantage is taken of the individual's need to 'make sense' of their experience and to attain consistency between themselves and their peer professionals. Utilising the work of Katz (1960) we can see how the occupational socialisation process and the function that attitudes serve the individual dovetail together, effective and complementary partners in crime.

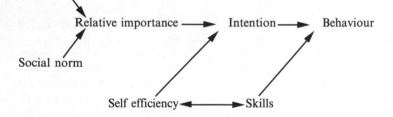

Fig. 2.3 Adapted model explaining the contribution of self-efficiency to intentional behaviour

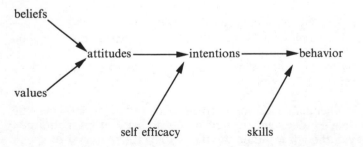

Fig. 2.4 Adapted model demonstrating the contribution which self efficacy may make

Attribution theories identify rules and biases that guide the individual in their sense-making of the behaviour they observe. These culture-specific interpretations become contextualised over time enabling the individual to understand and predict the attitudes, values and beliefs held in the professional environment.

Attitudes are learned. They can be learned tacitly or through open dialogue with ourselves (self-monitoring) or with others. The developing emphasis upon professional growth (PREPP) and professional practice being research-based and reflexive to client care contexts provides a forum for such a dialogue. The inevitable growth of self-awareness and self-empowerment may contribute to the quality of professional care. Leaving behind tacit ritual and routine.

With the current concerns to respond to the multi cultural health needs of the population, the change in the traditional profile of health care practitioners, and the changing context for health care provision, a partnership with dialogue will inevitably encourage sharing of attitudes, values and beliefs. This sharing has the potential then to facilitate choice, with awareness of those attitudes, values and beliefs the individual selects to adopt and aspire to.

References
Ajzen, I. and Fishbein, M. (1980). *Understanding Attitudes and Predicting Social Behavior*. Prentice-Hall, Englewood Cliffs.

Allport, G.W. (1954). *The Nature of Prejudice*. Addison Wesley, Reading.

Allport, G.W., Vernon, P. and Lindzey, G. (1970). *Manual for the Study of Values*, 3rd edn. Houghton-Mifflin, Boston.

Argyris, C. and Schön, D. (1974). *Theory in Practice*: *Increasing Professional Effectiveness*. Addison Wesley, Reading.

Argyris, C. and Schon, D. (1978). *Organizational Learning*: *a Theory of Action Perspective*. Addison Wesley, Reading.

Aronson, E. and Mills, J. (1959). The effect of severity of initiation on liking for a group. *Journal of Abnormal and Social Psychology*, 59, 177–81.

Atkinson, R.L., Atkinson, R.C., Smith, E.E. and Bem, D.J. (1990). *Introduction to Psychology*, 10th edn. Harcourt Brace Jovanovich, San Diego.

Atkinson, R.C. and Shiffrin, R.M. (1977). Human memory: a proposed system and its control processes. In *Human Memory*: *Basic Processes*, G.H. Bower (ed.). Academic Press, New York.

Bandura, A. (1977a). *Social Learning Theory*. Prentice-Hall, Englewood Cliffs.

Bandura, A. (1977b). Self efficacy: toward a unifying theory of behavioral change. *Psychological Review*, **84**, 191–215.

Bandura, A. (1986). *Social Foundation of Thought and Action*: *a Social-Cognitive Theory*. Prentice-Hall, Englewood Cliffs.

Bandura, A., Ross, D. and Ross, S.A. (1961). Transmission of aggression through imitation of aggressive models. *Journal of Abnormal and Social Psychology*, **63**, 575–87.

Bem, D.J. (1967). Self-perception: an alternative interpretation of cognitive dissonance phenomena. *Psychological Review*, **74**, 183–200.

Bem, D.J. (1972). Self-perception theory. In *Advances in Experimental Social Psychology. Volume 6*, L.D. Berkowitz (Ed.). Academic Press, New York.

Berger, P. and Luckman, T. (1966). *The Social Construction of Reality: a Treatise in the Sociology of Knowledge*. Anchor Books, New York.

Boud, D., Keogh, R. and Walker, D. (eds) (1985). *Reflection: Turning Experience into Learning*. Kogan Page, London.

Bradby, M. (1990). Status passage into nursing. *Journal of Advanced Nursing*, **15(10)**, 1220–5.

Broadbent, D.E. (1958). *Perception and Communication*. Pergamon, Oxford.

Burns, R.B. (1980). *Essential Psychology*. MTP, Lancaster.

Buss, A.R. (1979). *A Dialectical Psychology*. Invington, New York.

Caplan, G. (1974). *Support Systems and Mental Health*. Behavioral Publications, New York.

Cobb, S. (1976). Social support as a moderator of life stress. *Psychosomatic Medicine*, **38**, 300–14.

Cohen, S. and Wills, T.A. (1985). Stress, social support and the buffering hypothesis. *Psychological Bulletin*, **98**, 310–57.

Conway, M.E. (1983). Socialization and roles in nursing. *Annual Review of Nursing Research*, **1**, 183–208.

Crocker, L.M. and Brodie, B.J. (1974). Development of a scale to assess student nurses' views of one professional role. *Journal of Applied Psychology*, **59**, 233–5.

Davis, B.D. (1990). How nurses learn and how to improve the learning environment. *Nurse Education Today*, **10(6)**, 405–9.

de Vries, H., Dijkstra, M. and Kuhlman, P. (1988). Self-efficacy: the third factor beside attitude and subjective norm as a predictor of behavioral intentions. *Health Education Research*, **3(3)**, 273–82.

Dobbs, K.K. (1988). The senior preceptorship as a method for anticipatory socialization of baccalaureate nursing students. *Journal of Nursing Education*, **27(4)**, 167–71.

Dotan, M., Krulik, T., Bergman, R., Eckerling, S. and Shatzman, H. (1986). Occasional Paper. Role models in nursing. *Nursing Times*, **82(7)**, 55–7.

Erikson, E.H. (1968). *Identity: Youth and Crisis*. Faber, London.

Feldman, K.A. and Newcomb, T.M. (1969). *Impact of College on Students* Jossey Bass, San Francisco.

Festinger, L. (1957). *A Theory of Cognitive Dissonance*. Harper & Row, New York.

Festinger, L. and Carlsmith, J.M. (1959), Cognitive consequences of forced compliance *Journal of Abnormal and Social Psychology*, **58**, 203–10.

Fishbein, M. and Ajzen, I. (1975). *Belief, Attitude, Intention and Behavior Addison Wesley, Reading*.

Fiske, S.T. and Linville, P.W. (1980). What does the Schema concept buy us? *Personality and Social Psychology Bulletin*, **6(4)**, 543–57.

Glaser, B. and Strauss, A.L. (1971). *Status Passage*. Routledge and Kegan Paul, London.

Gross, R.D. (1987). *Psychology: the Science of Mind and Behaviour*. Hodder & Stoughton, London.

Gross, R.D. (1990). *Key Studies in Psychology*. Hodder & Stoughton, London.

Hagerty, B. (1986). A second look at mentors: do you really need one to suceed in nursing? *Nursing Outlook*, **34(1)**, 16–9, 24.

Hebb, D.O. (1949). *The Organization of Behaviour*. Wiley, New York.

Heider, F. (1958). *The Psychology of Interpersonal Relations*. Wiley, New York.

Hewstone, M. (1983). Attribution theory and common sense explanations: an introductory overview. In *Attribution Theory: Social and Functional Extensions*, M. Hewstone (ed.). Blackwell, Oxford.

Hilbert, G.A. and Allen, L.R. (1985). The effect of social support on educational outcomes. *Journal of Nursing Education*, **24(2)**, 48–52.

Homans, G.C. (1961). *Social Behaviour*: Its Elementary Forms. Harcourt Brace, New York.

Jones, E.E. and Davis, K.E. (1965). From acts to dispositions: the attribution process in social perception. In *Advances in Experimental Social Psychology Volume 2*, L. Berkowitz (ed.). Academic Press, New York.

Jones, H.D. (1982). Supervision: an educational process. In *Skills in Social and Educational Caring*, J.H. McMaster, (ed.). Gower, Aldershot.

Katz, D. (1960). The functional approach to the measures of attitudes. *Public Opinion Quarterly*, **24**, 163–204.

Kelley, H.H. (1967). Attribution theory in social psychology. In *Nebraska Symposium on Motivation. Volume 15*, D. Levine (ed.). University of Nebraska Press, Lincoln.

Kemper, T.D. (1968). Reference groups, socialization and achievement. *American Social Review*, **33**, 31–4.

Kilmann, R.H. (1981). Toward a unique/useful concept of values for interpersonal behavior: a critical review of the literature on value. *Psychological Reports*, **48**, 939–59.

Kramer, M. (1974). *Reality Shock*. Mosby, St Louis.

Kramer, M. and Schmalenberg, C. (1977). *Path to Biculturalism*. Wakefield Contemporary Publishing.

La Piere, R.T. (1934). Attitudes versus actions. *Social Forces*, **13**, 230–7.

Lent, R.H. and Hackett, G.C (1987). Career self efficacy: empirical status and future directions. *Journal of Vocational Behavior,* **30(3)**, 347–82.

Louis, M.R. (1980). Surprise and sense making: what newcomers experience in entering unfamiliar organizational settings. *Administrative Science Quarterly*, **25**, 226–51.

Maslow, A.H. (1987). *Motivation and Personality*, 3rd edn. Harper & Row. New York.

McGuire, W.J. (1969). The nature of attitudes and attitude change. In *Handbook of Social Psychology. Volume 3*, G. Lindzey and E. Aronson (eds). Addison-Wesley, Reading.

Melia, K. (1987). *Learning and Working the Occupational Socialization of Nurses*. Tavistock, London.

Menzies, I.E.P. (1970). *The Functioning of Social Systems as a Defence Against Anxiety*. Tavistock Institute of Human Relations, London.

Merron, K. (1957). *Social Theory and Social Structure*. Free Press, New York

Neidermeyer, E. and Neidermeyer, A.A. (1986). Employee motivation in a hospital *Journal of Nursing Administration*, **16(1)**, 12, 16.

Newcomb, T.M. (1950). *Social Psychology*. Dryden, New York.

Nisbett, R.E. and Ross, L. (1980). *Human Inference: Strategies and Shortcomings of Social Judgment*.

Olsson, H.M. and Gullberg, M.T. (1988). Nursing education and importance of professional status in the nurse's role: expectations and knowledge of the nurse role. *International Journal of Nursing Studies*, **25(4)**, 287–93.

O'Neill, M. (1975). A study of nursing student values. *International Journal of Nursing Studies*, **12(3)**, 175–81.

Osgood, C.E. and Tannenbaum, P.H. (1955). The principle of congruity in the prediction of attitude change. *Psychological Review*, **62**, 42–55.

Pennington, D.C. (1986). *Essential Social Psychology*. Edward Arnold,

Puetz, B.E. (1985). Learn the ropes from a mentor. *Nursing Success Today*, **2(6)**, 11–3.

Reber, A.S. (ed.) (1985). *The Penguin Dictionary of Psychology*. Penguin, Harmondsworth.

Rokeach, N. (1973). *The Nature of Human Values*. Free Press, New York.

Salvage, J. (1985). *The Politics of Nursing*. Heinemann, London.

Sarason, I.G. and Sarason, B.R. (Editors) (1985). *Social Support: Theory, Research and Applications*. Martinus Nijhoff

Schon, D. (1983). *The Reflective Practione*r Basic Books, New York.

Secord, P.F. and Backman, C.W. (1964). *Social Psychology*. McGraw-Hill, Auckland.

Sedhom, L.N. (1982). Attitudes toward the elderly among female college students. *Image*, **14(3)**, 81–5.

Shorter Oxford English Dictionary (1973) 3rd edn. Clarendon Press, Oxford.

Shuval, J.T. and Adler, I. (1980). The role of models in professional socialisation. *Social Science and* Medicine **14(1)**, 5–14.

Snyder, B.R. (1971). *The Hidden Curriculum*. MIT Press, Cambridge, Mass

Tedeschi, J.T., Schlenker, B.R. and Bonoma, T.V. (1971). Cognitive dissonance: private ratiocination or public spectacle. *American Psychologist*, **26**, 685–95.

United Kingdom Central Council for Nursing, Midwifery and Health Visiting (1984). *Code of Professional Conduct*, 2nd edn. UKCC, London.

United Kingdom Central Council for Nursing, Midwifery and Health Visiting (1986). *Project 2000: a New Preparation for Practice*. UKCC, London.

United Kingdom Central Council for Nursing, Midwifery and Health Visiting (1990). *The Report of the Post-Registration Education and Practice Project*. U.K.C.C., London.

Wilkins, E.J. (1976). *An Introduction to Sociology*, 2nd edn. Macdonald & Evans, London.

3 A Sociologist's View: the handmaiden's theory

Introduction: professional ladder or drawbridge?

This chapter seeks to uncover nurses' social/institutional roles in health care. The key to understanding why nurses carry out caring as they do, lies not in professed organisational intentions but within the depths of the hidden social structure. A sociologist's account of the hidden agenda in organised nursing sets out to answer three fundamental questions:

1. What is it in practice?
2. How does it affect nurses' roles in health?
3. Why do sociologists theorize about it in terms of winners and losers?

The hidden agenda may be defined as all the social learning that takes place in institutions outside the formally stated educational or occupational objectives. This social learning or adaptation to a role and its status location is called socialisation. It is an informal and largely unrecognised part of life in all social institutions.

In addition to *de jure* rules of conduct, which have been likened to a scientific version of the Ten Commandments (Becher, 1989; p. 27), workers have to familiarize themselves with the *de facto* or informal rules governing practices. While the *de jure* rules are constantly reiterated, these may bear no relation to the way the work is actually accomplished. While the *de facto* rules may account realistically for work practices, these are not defined or explained. Subordinate workers, and this includes nurses, have a real problem. They have to make the work prescriptions of higher occupations a reality – but what version of reality? Whose knowledge is the 'right' interpretation? 'You are not here to think, Nurse!' is a likely response to requests for clarification. Confronted with such perplexity, it is hardly surprising that many people resort to pragmatism: 'I'll just have to work it out on my own.' Collective frustrations, which are the result of competitive ways of working, are experienced as personalised problems and not as the consequences of a disadvantaged position.

The handmaiden mentality and tasks of nurses are not natural female responses to human need or male technical superiority. They are the outcome of a system which openly supports separations between cure and care, while covertly relying upon nurses to fill the gap in between. Nurses are used to fit the spaces where one technical job ends and another begins. So-called normal practices rely upon nurses to exceed the scope of their official job responsibilities.

In the development of hospital medicine, the destinies of doctors and nurses have been closely linked. The first group, however, has an established and prestigious place in health; the latter do not. In the sociology of the professions, this is a constructed dominance on the part of medicine which necessitates the impoverishment of para-medical and semi-professional groups (Freidson, 1970). Professionals have the strength and power to exclude others, to weaken their claims. Unequal exchange, and the degree of inter-dependency between occupations on the professional 'ladder', are not always acknowledged in health organisation. Formal systems expect uniformity in response, operating on a basis of an assumed consensus, thereby denying real separations in their ranks based upon occupational power, gender or ethnicity.

Health professionalism is not a 'ladder' but a hierarchy or pyramid of power. Different groups have differing views depending on their location and access to decision-making processes; the open agenda. For doctors, dentists or research chemists, the view from the top is a plurality of competing interest groups trying to dislodge medicine from the pinnacle. The view of those near the bottom is one of a fairly rigid structure, unsupportive of their needs, with clear boundaries of authority and skill between those who have the power to decide and those who do not. This is the normality for the majority of nurses in health care.

The contrasting experiences of occupational groups is the consequence of their relationship to each other in the formal hierarchy. While those in the higher ranks may use the power of their position to make the rules as they go along, others have to obey the changing 'orders of the day'. Nurses receive instructions in obedience beyond stated objectives relating to their roles as organisational agents. Nurses serve, not an abstract entity called health organisation, but the interests of real people with a superior status. This constitutes nursing's hidden agenda. According to sociologists, the legitimate or open system of authority can too easily become a rationale of compliance for all those excluded from leadership roles: 'Control from the top needs to be reciprocated by discipline from the bottom'. (Bauman 1990; p. 81).

Hierarchy was originally a system of military government in the Roman Empire whereby the army was organised into a pyramid of ranks and subject to standard rules and procedures; the 'War Machine' of imperial Rome. The contemporary meaning includes any organisation whose members or employees are arranged in a status order of rank, grade or class. In popular usage it is taken to be a denigrating feature of large-scale bureaucracies and government institutions. All change is official, emanating from the top. Modern bureaucracies resemble the original hierarchy in that the competence of an employee is determined not by outsiders but by his/her superiors in the hierarchy. Consequently, everything subordinate groups do tends to be used to promote their superiors and not themselves.

Nurses, especially trainees, suffer from this officialdom in that they are treated like mushrooms and 'kept in the dark'. Communication tends to be restricted to a need-to-know basis; the rule of secret sessions. Nursing as an occupation is overshadowed by medical professionalism. But it is overseen by an industrial or business mentality of expediency embodied in classic managerialism. Health bureaucracies make hidden demands upon nurses to conform, despite official claims to nursing's honorary professional status. Consequently, nurses may be unaware of their importance to higher status specialists rather than to patients.

The handmaiden problem in nursing: ladies or cleaning ladies?

What is unimportant and essential at the same time? The answer is nursing care within the prevailing social order in health. This paradox will be explored here in relation to nurses' largely hidden purposes. Nurses, used as a flexible workforce of professionally motivated carers, have important but unrecognised roles completing the tasks of patient care that others leave behind.

Unlike many specialists and technicians, nurses have interchangeable functions in health organisation. On the one hand, nurses are expected to act as deferential handmaidens to doctors and administrators. On the other, they are supposed to initiate and control patient care when these higher authorities are absent.

> in his absence [the doctor] will expect her to be able to make quite complex decisions relating to the patient's condition and care and to be able to initiate the appropriate action.
>
> (Chapman, 1976; p. 113)

Nurses have to be intelligent 'doers' but they must not expect full recognition for their inventiveness. Instead they receive, if good manners prevail, gratitude for an interest almost taken to be momentary. This ambiguous status is reflected in the tentative way nurses learn to report their observations, for instance, 'I was doing Mrs Jones' back and I happened to notice how restless/hot/cold she was'.

Nurses have a personal responsibility for patients' needs. This informal commitment may be contrasted with the specialisms of the experts, falling on the side of care while the process of cure appears to be a more elite province. Caring is defined as routine, physical work which denies its significance in patient recovery and medical cure. Nurses have conducted health care for a long time. Yet employers continue to treat nurses as if they were doing them a favour allowing them to participate in the technical process.

Nurses have paradoxical roles in health organisation. They are *marginal* to medical, scientific education and yet *central* to medical health practices. At the level of health provision, curative sciences are taken to be naturally superior and distinct from occupations and work groups directly involved in caring for people. Nursing care is a vital part of institutionalised medicine; the extent of its use to uphold the specialisms of higher status groups is not acknowledged in the open health agenda. The nature of nurses' social roles in service delivery remains something of a mystery, even to nurses themselves.

Nursing is not, contrary to popular belief, a natural female response to caring (see Chapter 1). Instead it is a socially organised occupation. Categorised as predominantly practical and female activity, nursing lies low in the occupational hierarchy of health professions. The vocational commitment many nurses bring to their work, the gifts of goodness and helping, may be essential to a patient's self-esteem and well-being. However, within a treatment system concerned primarily with acute care and rife with technological expertise, these nursing qualities are not seen to be very important to scientific progress. Consequently, in health provision nursing definitions of what is needed tend to be overlooked.

Nurses also have conflicting roles. Health administrators want self-disciplined domestic servants to carry out the patient's housework. Doctors require professionally educated nurses to implement their treatment prescriptions with care and precision. Nurses' public service ethic requires them to put the needs of patients for independence before their own personal or occupational needs. At the same time, nurses are supposed to pursue a strategy of professionalism which means securing their occupational interests on the organisational agenda. 'To be or not to be honorable cleaning ladies, or lady professionals?' This is a serious question confronting modern nursing, nor is it just a nursing problem. The way nursing care is labelled and undervalued in health as a type of domesticated, personal service is linked to the de-valuing of caring, spirituality and practical work in society generally. These processes are the result, as we shall see, of deeply rooted social prejudices such as class and gender.

There is much discussion in nursing about the low status of caring in the bio-medical or hospital model. Nursing care is not complementary to medical cure, it is subordinate. This care/cure distinction is not a natural but a social construction, almost a mythology. It is not, however, the fault of nurses. The handmaiden's role is not one that nurses have chosen for themselves.

Anti-intellectualism in nursing is not the cause but the effect of its subservient status in health organisation (See Chapter 1). Nurses have not gained control over the creative or qualitative aspects of their work. Medical and health authorities in a public or private service evaluate and regulate nursing's mental horizons and objective conditions. An analysis of nursing's hidden agenda is not confined to its internal ranking order, ideology of altruistic service, methods of education or supervision. The approach here suggests a wider, institutional framework; the behavioural expectations and system of rules bind nurses, not necessarily to their patients' needs, but to the interests of powerful groups within the health industry.

Intimate relations: the open and hidden agenda

The hidden agenda in nursing, viewed through the sociological lens, is the consequence of its subordinate place in social medical institutions. Nurses are charged with the responsibility to carry out the orders of others without the authority to affect major structural decisions concerning modes of practice. Nursing outcomes may be described as the following experiences:

1. Being treated like a pair of hands or feet and not as an intelligent adult.
2. Carrying out the orders of authority figures without knowing the reasons why.
3. Not being allowed to talk to patients because this might reveal medical information nurses and patients are not entitled to have.
4. Sympathising with the needs of those in authority to the detriment of nurses' needs and those of the patients'.
5. Being skilled, confident and flexible enough to clean up the mess left by other groups when they go home after a day's work.
6. Taking the unpaid and unrecognised responsibility for patients' personal needs; thus 'freeing' the specialists to pursue the status of their positions and keep control over methods of care.

The hidden agenda is not a random side-effect or marginal issue confined to nursing practice or nursing education (see Chapter 4). Instead it is an integral part of nursing's long history of subservience to hospital medicine and hospital administration (see Chapter 1). The consequence for nurses is an inferior status in their institutional roles compared to that of their professional or idealized nursing model. The old problem of powerlessness in nursing cannot be cured by assertiveness training, quality management styles or even an academic education. Nurses' lack of authority is not the fault of passive individuals but a system of health care which undervalues caring as non-scientific work.

The less control an occupation may exercise over its practices, the more likely members' needs will remain 'invisible' at the level of formal organisation. Nursing's position in the health hierarchy or pyramid of power, tends more towards an imposed dependency than control. This means that a large amount of nursing activity comes into the area of informal practices; constituting the hidden agenda. Much of the social learning of routines and procedures that nurses, particularly trainees, experience in adjusting to institutional life, is not openly acknowledged as an essential part of the job. Health institutions, therefore, make harsh demands upon nurses which they must resolve in individual ways.

The consequences of this in terms of know-how knowledge in nursing, I see as a tragedy. A considerable amount of first-hand knowledge, gained from a history of hands-on care, is either passed from senior to junior staff in an *ad hoc* fashion or lost forever. Not all trial and error learning, customary practices or intuition are necessarily detrimental to safe and healthy practices. The reason this nursing mentality has remained, until recently, in obscurity and the reason it continues to be low status, even in nursing, is the dominance of the curative model in health care. The mentality of caring is submerged within medicine's empirical science based upon doctors' experiences of illness and not that of patients or carers. Sick people need and respond to care. Caring enhances the achievements of expert health workers, in particular, the famous couple relationship between doctor and patient. It is a subject worthy of independent study (Jolley and Brykczyńska, 1992).

At present nurses and their caring do not have a status independent of the institutional medical model. When nurses attempt to treat patients as people, they tend to get into trouble. For example, talking to patients is not considered to be nurses' work. The patient's integrity is sacrificed to management directives to get the work done as quickly as possible. More importantly, talking to patients implies building up a personal relationship whereby nurses might inadvertently criticise the doctor's way of treating the patient.

> whilst nurses have opinions, there is no place for their expression in the workplace. In order for patients to believe and continue to believe that doctors are omniscient and omnipotent, they must not see anyone expressing disagreement with a doctor's judgement. The doctor's image must be upheld.
>
> (Keddy et al., 1986; p. 749)

The majority of practitioners may be mystified by the version of nursing emanating from their professional associations and teachers. Their reality is shaped more by factory logic or production line techniques, and classic over-seeing management rather than any concept of altruism or advocacy. Their work involves 'making do' and 'cutting corners' without knowing why certain tasks take precedence over others. Melia's (1987) research on nurse trainees refers to this as 'working in the dark'. No wonder many nurses define their roles not in professional terms but as organisational imperatives. Despite the nursing theory of holistic caring it is apparent that real barriers to this approach exist in health organisation.

Hidden agendas reveal that social institutions have different ways of valuing people apart from openly stated rules and socially acceptable means. There may be a vast area of experience and expertise which is not recognised by an organisation or its value-system as real or really important. This could mean a denial of a considerable amount of work. For nurses, this is the commitment they bring to their caring. Personalised caring is time-consuming, labour-intensive, creative and concerned with a patient's self-definition of need; hence it is expensive and political. Far better that it remain, at present, invisible in health institutions thus perpetuating the dependency of nurses and clients on scientific measurements of need, and not their own definitions.

Open agendas are the organisation's plans for action and lists of items to be acted upon according to agreed priorities and the desired quality of the product; whether goods, services or human beings. The open agenda in health is efficiency and higher quality care, carried out by motivated people in teams, groups and occupations. Individuals holding roles within the hierarchy have to mould themselves to fit predetermined functions. At the same time the organisation requires a high level of flexibility to enable the workforce to respond to everyday problems which arise. This is where nurses and helper groups, as wide-ranging generalists, have a key role to play in the delivery of care.

Organisational flexibility stems overtly from a well-qualified and hand-picked workforce where possible, and covertly, from the diverse pool of personal skills, talents and life experiences which many adults bring to their learning in education or work. At the covert level, unacknowledged personal expertise emerges; for example, who is best at doing what? This enables a certain amount of personal development which is denied by the rigid, formal system of credentialism or paper qualifications. It could be the main reason a ward or day centre continues to function efficiently, despite chronic under-funding and under-staffing. But it can also mean that nobody gets to learn something they do not feel confident about! This was, and is a real problem for nurses within an apprenticeship training scheme.

Open agendas impose roles and regulated activities, but leave the substance of the work to the realm of informal or negotiated relations. However, the degree of inter-dependency between individuals and groups, needed to get all the work accomplished, is vastly underestimated. Although labour is supposedly rationally or functionally divided, that is, impersonal, in reality every person's job is mediated by another's. The order of the day may be the 'rule of routine' or the scientific formula, but this conceals a tangled web of interpersonal actions which may be crucial to the running of the organisation.

While the open agenda in organisations defines the existing authority structure, the use of the hidden agenda is to defend it. In other words, stated aims are carried through by largely unstated means to ensure compliance to the 'business-in-hand'. Practitioners have to contend with inconsistencies or double standards, dual roles and divided selves. For example, nurses are expected to be pragmatists but in a different situation to act as self-reliant, risk-taking real professionals. The result of this duality is the trade-off, or the constant bargaining and bickering over who is responsible for what. Who is going to end up 'giving in' and agreeing to the compliant role when so many want to be the equivalent of the doctor (Heenan, 1990)? Crisis management appears to be inevitable because 'for every institutional norm . . . one can find at least one counter norm prescribing a diametrically opposed line of action.' (Merton, 1973 in Becher, 1989; P. 26)

These are frustrating, organisational problems but people are left to find their own solutions on the basis of, 'Other people seem to cope. why can't I?' For subordinate groups this frequently ends in tears, fears, guilt and anxiety. It is usually measured in terms of higher rates of occupational stress, absenteeism, illness and attrition.

> Initial investigation of nurse recruitment and wastage demonstrated that the 'problem' was not why nurses left, but why given the often appalling conditions under which they work, they stayed. The health authority's 'problem' was nurse' 'solution' to difficult and demanding work environments.
>
> (Mackay, 1990; P. 29)

Nurses, like other direct producers, acquire the values and patterns of behaviour expected of them the 'hard way', largely through their on-the-job experiences. But they learn more than just *how* to do their work; they must also *know their place*. The consequences are identified in nursing as the imposition of task-centred care, and in social research as the imposition of rules and meanings to ensure obedience. Nurses have to reconcile the conflict between their ideal of health care and the reality of trying to negotiate the clinical environment (Ho, 1989; P. 291).

Professional codes of practice value good nurses in terms of compassion and care, while institutional values equate competence with behaviour which supports the rules, rituals, and status quo. Nurses have to adjust to their humble place in the health hierarchy through the process of meeting the expectations of powerful groups within the organisation. An important part of their occupational socialisation is the constant enactment of ceremonies of power to reinforce existing inequalities. Obvious examples in hospital nursing are first, the doctor-nurse game (Stein, et al. 1990) and secondly, the labelling of the unpopular patient (Stockwell, 1972). These are only two examples of taken-for-granted rites in nursing, arising out of a hospital tribalism or culture (Strong and Robinson, 1988).

In this discussion, nursing as an occupation is viewed as an imposed rather than a negotiated order. Nurses' roles are not defined by the status of those performing the tasks, but are confirmed as low status to begin with. To take account of this institutional power, I have defined the hidden agenda as

> the routine practices, traits of behaviour and even unconscious motivation used in human interaction, acquired through participation in organised groups, and the significance of these processes to existing power relations.

The five sociological dimensions mentioned in this definition are described in Table 3.1. These provide the main themes for an analysis of occupational experiences within the informal social structure. Applied to nursing, the following picture emerges.

Table 3.1 Hidden Agenda in nursing: sociological dimensions (learning your place)

Hidden social processes	Consequences for nurses: occupational socialisation	Uses in the health order: imposed social roles
1. Routine practices (not necessarily unseen but unexplained)	Task-centred care: bending the rules to get the work completed on time. Nurses extend the scope of their caring responsibilities	Nurses are used interchangeably as generalists. They fill the spaces where one job technically ends and another begins
2. Traits of behaviour	Acquired deference to any authority figure, even those whose rank only just exceeds one's own (saluting the 'uniform' not the person who wears it)	Nurses learn to handle the egos of those in authority-sustains the belief in leadership. The authority structure appears undisturbed
3. Unconscious motivation or self-serving interests	The pursuit of careers by individuals, work groups or occupations takes precedence over professional standards. Promotion takes place on the basis of preferment and privilege, not overt indicators or merit	Nurses must resolve in personal ways, tensions between their own need for independance and patient-centred care. Nurses' lack of status and esteem is seen to be a purely nursing problem

4. Participation in the status organised groups	Nurses 'learn the ropes' and in the process come to terms with the conflicts between nursing values and the imperatives of service delivery	Nurses acquired mentality which corresponds to their subordinate place in the health hierarchy. Existing inequalities are maintained
5. Covert power or structural autonomy over nursing practices	Control of nursing by those with a monopoly to decide how caring takes place. Caring is defined as menial work and carers have an inferior status	Nurses are used as handmaidens to uphold technical specialism. Existing divisions between cure and care are maintained. Nurses project discontent on to each other and not the politics and policies of health organisation as a whole

Normal concepts of 'good' and 'bad' used in nursing are not, therefore, solely derived from its formal structure and professional intentions. In fact, the open agenda may be largely a myth which workers are usually aware of. For instance, a recent newspaper article on guidelines to success in office work stated:

> Offices live by myths – it is necessary to work hard and complete certain tasks – which have nothing to do with reality. The reality is bravura displays of self-promotion. Ambitious young people are advised to ignore their jobs and think about how to flatter and cajole people in power to give them a better job.
>
> (Bedell, G., 1992)

All occupations are therefore something of a mystery unless you are 'one of the gang'. Nurses are supposed to develop in certain ways but the appropriate behaviour is not clearly stated. They are meant to portray deferential attitudes to everyone, yet be prepared at all times to take the initiative and stand up for patients' rights. They have to acquire particular forms of knowledge but no one tells them what it is. They have to make contact with certain people so that the work gets done but no one tells them who to turn to. Trainee staff, passing from ward to ward, are at a particular disadvantage. They have to establish themselves anew each time they encounter a ward's permanent staff who have their own ways of working.

> As a new student on the ward you really get depressed because . . . even before you begin to think about the patients and how you are going to treat the patients – you begin to think 'just as long as I settle into the ward, get on with the staff'. That's the most important thing. You become two-faced, really, you're doing things . . . just to get on with the staff.
>
> (Melia, 1984; p. 141)

Nurses work in large-scale, bureaucratic organisations where power is concentrated at the top, stifling any questioning of the in-house authority.

Unlike more powerful groups who make the rules, nurses have a meticulous responsibility to carry them out. Nurses are vulnerable to abuses of power which have become known as adult 'bullying at work'.

> Bullying is the misuse of power, the misuse of position to intimidate somebody in a way which leaves them feeling very hurt, vulnerable, angry and impotent.
>
> (Crawford, 1991, quoted in Adams, 1991)

It usually comes in a number of disguises. Here are some examples which you may be familiar with in your place of work:

1. *A personality clash*: blocking another staff member's promotion.
2. *Poor management style*: refusal to delegate.
3. *Aggression*: rages over 'trivial' matters.
4. *Intimidation*: persistent criticism.
5. *Harrassment*: inflicting menial tasks.
6. *Autocratic management*: removing areas of responsibility.
7. *Working in an 'idiosyncratic' or 'funny' way*: talking only to a third party to isolate another.
8. *Unreasonable behaviour*: personal insults.

(Adams, 1991).

The consequences may be *seen*, such as shouting at members of staff or *unseen*, for example, turning down leave requests for no discernible reason. These are all aspects of behaviour associated with organisational hidden agendas. The sorting of the winners from the losers is conveniently shunted onto individuals on the basis of: 'Let them sort it out themselves'.

The agenda is an organisation's plans for action or the business in hand. This is a dictionary definition. If we look up agenda in *Roget's Thesaurus* (1962) where words are grouped not alphabetically but according to meaning, a more realistic picture emerges. Starting with benign meanings such as 'order of the day' and 'transactions', I was led to 'irons in the fire' and 'axes to grind' and came across pathological tendencies such as connivance and conspiracy. An understanding of agenda implies moving from openly professed incentives to very hidden, manipulative control of organisational resources by powerful, self-serving individuals or groups. Organisations have manifest functions which may be understood even if not agreed as well as latent functions or hidden intentions which to many people may be as 'clear as mud' (Giddens, 1989; p. 697).

Organisations are set up and government-funded with a socially acceptable purpose. But in reality those involved in setting up the organisation and those working within it have their own interests and seek to pursue their own purposive activities within the system. These interests and self-serving activities are unlikely to be socially approved or government-funded since they are to benefit the individual rather than serve the public. These aims are part of the hidden agenda.

When a proposal is made by an individual which would be of benefit to him/herself, the actor seeks to justify the proposition or sell the idea as being of benefit to society. Adam Smith, a classical economist, has pointed out, that in order to sell your meat, you speak not of your needs but of the hunger of your client. The greater the discrepancy between the benefits to the proposer and those to the client, disguised by a jargon of justification, the more we may speak of the hidden agenda.

For example, the dentist will say that the most important part of health care is dentistry. Opticians are very forward in telling us the value of eye tests for all age-groups. Opticians are paid every time they look into our eyes, and dentists every time they look into our mouths, and we are grateful for their interest. This is a hidden economic incentive in health service professionalism.

In order to illustrate this movement from an organisation's professed mission of public service to 'invisible' self-interest, I have categorised informal control and work incentives on a scale of concealment, extending from seen use to unseen use of an institution's public trust. The higher the number the greater the misuse of authority. This is my own version. Readers may find they need to rearrange the points on the scale between the two extremes to express their own occupational experiences.

First, we need to define the seven main behavioural categories. These are the personal costs in terms of imposed values and actions as shown below.

Hidden Agenda: behavioural categories

1. *Routine practices*: bending the rules or overcoming official constraints to get the work completed on time; covering for those who 'shrink' into their job description and do the minimum. These processes are seen but not necessarily accepted as explanations for the extra work.
2. *Extending role responsibilities*: taking care of patients' personal needs; nurses act as intermediaries between doctor and patient and as a buffer between the patient and the impersonality of a bureaucratic health service (Mackay 1989).
3. *Trade offs*: between individuals, work groups and occupations; finding out the contacts to be made in order to know what work is to be done, how to do it, and who is to be held responsible. Occupations transfer their dirty work to lower status groups/individuals.
4. *Intellectual seduction or willing compliance*: individuals know that if they follow-the-leader willingly, he/she will be promoted and then there will be a position vacant for them! Promotion is dependent upon securing the preferment of the authority figure rather than any indicator of merit. This requires members of staff to ignore their peers and concentrate on their usefulness to superiors. The emphasis is on identifying with a career and not professional values (public service).
5. *Bullying or unwilling compliance*: public or private shaming, humiliation or constant criticism, such as being treated as pairs of hands or feet; trained nurses are used interchangeably with auxiliary staff (Melia, 1987).
6. *Connivance or scheming*: preventing others from obtaining the information they need to get their work done, for example simply not telling someone that an important meeting is to take place, or not passing on information

about changes in a patient's condition and treatment – consequently those 'picked on' get into trouble. At the same time, the schemer will take all the credit for any good work done by others.

7. *Conspiracy or betrayal of people's trust*: lying to patients or their relatives in their 'best interests'; participating in cover-ups to disguise the lack of proper care or even malpractice. Blocking a person's promotion for personal reasons – they are likely to do the job better!

These categories are expressed in Fig. 3.1 on a scale of concealment: informal controls and incentives in work, the informal hierarchy. These act as barriers to the enactment of nursing roles.

As stated above, readers may wish to devise their own categories relevant to their experiences. I would maintain the two end points of (1) routine bending of the rules and (7) conspiracy, the hidden agenda in its extreme form.

While the open agenda is socially acceptable, it might not be if its hidden consequences were revealed. Many tensions and conflicts arising out of competitive ways of working and assessing individuals, which is the institutional order, may be evaded by relegation to the hidden agenda. Overall functioning appears to be consensual and undisturbed. Individuals are not rewarded or supported according to the difficulties they face in trying to get their work done. These processes are always linked, according to sociologists, to some form of power and social inequity.

Relations of power are some of society's best-kept secrets. These processes are part of the everyday world and they hardly warrant discussion. However, any resistance is likely to be labelled as unreasonable behaviour, deviance or outright lunacy! This can amount to the suppression of free speech. For instance, when doctors or nurses voice concern about their patients' unmet needs, they may be severely censored. In recent years we have seen the case of Wendy Savage, a consultant obstetrician, who was taken to court for promoting natural childbirth practices in a London Hospital (Savage, 1986). Graham Pink, a nurse, voiced his worries about standards of care for the elderly. After much controversy and attacks on his personal integrity and professional competence, I believe he is now, at the time of writing, unemployed (Faugier, 1991). When staff appeal to their appropriate line managers to help solve problems of this kind, their concern may be dismissed or denigrated as a personal or mischievous complaint.

According to sociologists.

> Power not discussed is power taken for granted. The underlying assumption held consciously or not is that existing arrangements are fundamentally just, those who have power ought to have it and those who do not, should not.

> (Howton, 1969; p. 80)

Sociologists study the means by which oppression achieves the status of being normal, commonplace and socially acceptable, hence 'invisible'. In order for power to be used effectively, it is necessary that people feel the need for it is justified. In other words, members of 'down-trodden' groups have to believe in their own inferiority. The perpetuation of the social order in health, however, may not mean peace and consensus only an on-the-surface acceptance of the status quo. In order to survive in organisations one has to

> acquire the 'savoir faire' which consists in knowing how to handle . . . conflicting rules, when to invoke one and perhaps practise the other.
>
> (Becher, 1989; p. 27)

One moment the ward or unit operates on the hidden agenda: 'I don't care if it's not your job Nurse; the patient is your responsibility!' The next minute, the emphasis shifts to upholding the open authority structure: 'How dare you give advice to that patient Nurse: that is the doctor's responsibility!' It would appear from the recent production of books on politics in nursing that nurses do not agree that existing power relations in health are necessarily peaceful or justified (Robinson, 1991).

The handmaiden mentality: patient care

Professional caring philosophy with its accountability to the patient does not explain the subordinate place of nurses in health care. The nurse's role in the patient's right to health is taken for granted. Nursing is seen to be a health profession complementary to medical practice, attached to medicine like a semi-detached house. We do not learn where nurses' low status comes from; what variety of tasks they perform; how they can be responsible to patients when they do not have the authority to decide how caring takes place; what obstructions they face in trying to carry out personalised caring or why caring, a fundamental human prerequisite, has such a low value in health and society anyway. Meanwhile, nurses who use their professional code to assess patient care and find it wanting may face dire consequences if they speak out. Labelled as 'whistle blowers', these concerned carers are likely to find themselves rejected: 'Once an individual begins to make noises about unsafe practices or standards he or she is singled out as a trouble-maker.' (Turner, 1991; p. 20)

It is not the idea or ideology of professionalism which unifies nursing with all its diverse activities and meanings. Instead unity and status are constituted via a number of higher authorities, in particular, the Welfare State. Brought together as members of a welfare occupation, the status of nurses was raised at the inception of the National Health Service in 1948. More recent developments describe a career structure in terms of managerialism. To many clinical or community specialists, this may not be a career at all.

It is a pity that the handmaiden's complaints have never been developed into the handmaiden's theory. Nurses' roles continue to be described and analysed in terms of a professional interaction between the nurse and the patient. But the real relationship is, and has been, between nursing care and health administration.

Numerous issues confronting nursing are seen to stem from the theory/ practice divide in nursing or the education/service division in nursing or the professional caring versus the work ethic in nursing and the end result is *nurses*

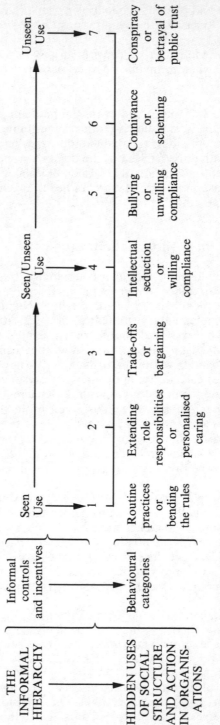

Fig. 3.1   Scale of Concealment: informal controls and incentives in work organisation

versus *nurses*. At the same time, very little is known about the relation of nurses to other nurses, the relation of nursing to medicine or nurses to the organisations in which they work. Nurses' role-obligations extend from an increasing number of conflicting interest-groups; for instance:

1. *Nurse-nurse*: the views of the majority of nurses may not coincide with those of their professional leadership.

   Nurses, midwives and health visitors may have different orientations to their caring work as a profession, vocation or just a job (Mackay, 1990).

   Midwives do not want to be seen as nurses but professionals equal in status to doctors (Ho, 1989).

   Nurses do not see health visitors as 'proper' nurses (Pearson and Vaughan, 1986).

   The majority of bedside or clinical care is carried out by the lowest status groups in the nursing hierarchy, e.g. state enrolled nurses and auxiliary staff (Melia, 1987).

2. *Nurse-doctor*: nursing actions are initiated by medical directives based upon the mechanistic and impersonal medical model. Nearly all approaches to patient care are mediated through clinical categories which means nurses are instrumental in socialising patients into the passive sick role (Perry, 1991).

   Nurses assert their understanding of the work doctors do, not an understanding of what *they* do or what patients' *want* (Jones, 1987).

3. *Nurse-organisation*: nurses' vocational ideology justifies their use as generalists; presumes that they will undertake as much work as is necessary (no matter how unpleasant) irrespective of rewards, status or control.

   Nurses are used as the tools of management's trade (White, 1988; p. 17).

At the same time nurses maintain an intense, formal and informal, responsiveness to patients' needs.

4. *Nurse-patient*: nurses are involved in face-to-face contact with patients – they are aware of patients' feelings and self-definitions of need. They relieve the 'experts' of a need to concern themselves with patients' fears. They carry out physical care when people are unable to do this themselves; this is an important aspect of a patient's recovery.

Nursing may be at least three semi-professions; a diversity which is reflected in the title of its foremost professional association, the United Kingdom Central Council for Nursing, Midwifery and Health Visiting. Nursing itself is not a homogeneous category but a hierarchy, the lowest grades carrying out the bulk of physical care. Sociologically, this has been viewed as an ethnic and class division.

> The three grades of nursing – auxiliaries, state enrolled and state registered – form a clear hierarchy with little or no possibility of training to move up the qualification hierarchy. Women from ethnic minorities are concentrated in the auxiliary and state enrolled grades,

and white middle-class women in the registered grade in the prestigious teaching hospitals.

(Abbott and Wallace, 1990a; p. 24)

The tensions arising from all these interacting, institutional roles and relationships tend to be relegated to the hidden agenda where they are viewed as personal complaints and not organisational problems. 'They call nursing the caring profession, but you know, who does care for the carers?' (Student Nurse, quoted in Mackay, 1989; p. 113). Nurses' place in health is not necessarily valued and judged in ways that make sense, especially to nurses patients or sociologists. The logic which informs and justifies the low status of nursing care is not the result of necessity (a human response to recognised health needs), but the logic of an industrial form of health provision.

Nurses are not employed in the health service to express themselves but to manufacture a system of caring. They do not work as independent professionals who may openly govern their own practices. The majority of nurses in the United Kingdom carry out caring within professional models largely defined by their employers. As a welfare occupation, nursing's main objective is to make the work prescriptions of higher status groups a reality. Since this organisational intention is never openly stated, it is hardly surprising that nurses remain confused about what their roles are. Their approaches to patients, that is, the mentality or quality of care, and the methods implemented are mediated through the powerful institutions of medicine and general health management. The consequence for nurses is a lack of authority to initiate caring actions in the self-defined interests of patients.

Roles are statuses-in-action. They are not neutral, all roles being relative to the status of those above and below in the ranking order. If a patient is not progressing as the doctor ordered, the vigilant nurse does not alter the treatment, she calls the doctor. This nurse knows her place. But what does she do when

1. A doctor's orders for medication are wrong, or
2. A doctor asks her to alter a patient's case notes and withhold information in the event of a complaint?

In the first case

> nurses agreed that a dilemma arose when they needed to criticize or question a physician's decision. Conflict often occurred when the medication orders written by physicians needed clarification, because dispensing medications is a legal and ethical nursing responsibility. Even if a physician prescribed a drug or dosage incorrectly or illegibly, a nurse would be legally liable for administrating it to a patient.

(Katzman and Roberts, 1988)

In the second case

> Deliberately altering a patient's case notes to falsify what events did or did not take place has serious repercussions for the patient. Nurses may

have to decide whether they should be the doctor's handmaiden or the patient's friend. They cannot be both.

(Robinson, 1986)

There may not be a '*white coat with a stethoscope in the pocket*' in sight. It is unlikely that a top administrator will appear on the ward or at the clinic or day centre. But these authorities are ever-present in the minds of nurses in terms of behavioural expectations and attitudes to patient care which govern nursing practices. These abstract social relationships are as powerful and real as any physical presence. For a trainee nurse or midwife, nurse and patient interaction is not a private consultation between a professional and a client. Instead, the nurse's responsibility to the patient is translated formally into institutional rules and standardised treatment procedures. (Covertly nurses maintain an intense responsiveness to patient need.) Nursing and caring are not defined according to a powerful professional role but a status viewed as a derivation from the norms of medical behaviour and technical cure.

> Nurses define their roles around and after medical diagnosis. The doctor decides who is to be a patient, where and for how long. He is held in higher esteem than the nurse. His work is more highly valued and certainly more highly paid.
>
> (Jones, 1987)

Formal or open agendas in organisations describe work role and occupation narrowly in terms of functions, leaving most of the work to be accomplished in substantive ways to largely informal processes (the hidden agenda). In health organisation, nurses are defined solely in terms of their *instrumental* caring functions. This means they are treated like pairs of hands and pairs of feet. Within this organisational context, imaginative nursing care becomes dramatically reduced to technical competencies carried out by qualified staff, and routine physical tasks allocated to trainees and helpers. Similarly, a patient's suffering unique to each individual, becomes reduced to a commonplace case of this or that clinical condition. Is this all there is to caring and to the patient's suffering? The answer is simply, 'no'.

Caring fills the time and space available because high standards combined with an infinite variety of individual human needs make it diverse and *endless*. As mentioned earlier, nurses are used in health care covertly as highly skilled generalists. They clean up the mess other occupations and work groups leave behind. They fill the spaces where one job or specialist occupation ends and another begins. Nurses must carry out medicine's dirty work with intelligence and vigilance. Because nursing is a licentiate health profession they have to do this according to their own high standards. Their personal responsibility for patients, their vocation, means they must see that all the necessary tasks of patient care are accomplished, even when the work is not, officially, their own.

Nurses tend to work everywhere in health, for generalised patient care is not confined to a specific area. As a consequence they may feel personally responsible for standards throughout the whole health service. While other occupations may pursue self-interest, nurses must put the needs of patients before their own needs for independence and status. While these social uses of nurses in health continue to be covertly controlled by higher status authorities, many practitioners may not be aware of their importance to other occupations rather than to their clients.

Nursing care as a function of health organisation is not seen to be an essential quality related to a patient's recovery or even cure, but merely a list of routine tasks imposed by more powerful occupations. When nurses carry out a complex procedure such as administering medication to a patient, it becomes a routine drug round. When they act responsibly in the dramas of operating theatres, intensive care units, or prevent a patient knowingly injuring him or herself, they are working according to this or that set of routine, emergency procedures. Even when, through sheer competence and resourcefulness, they recognise that a patient is showing signs of entering a crisis, they have to pretend they do not fully understand the implications of the situation when reporting to the doctor. They must resort to playing the doctor-nurse game (Stein, 1967). In order to get the patient's needs met, they must know how to adroitly handle the egos of those with medical authority.

> In 1967 there was clear agreement between doctors and nurses that their relationship was hierarchical, with doctors being superior to nurses. All their interactions were carefully managed so as not to disturb the hierarchy. Nurses were to be bold, have initiative and be responsible for making important recommendations, while at the same time they had to appear passive. In short, nurses were to make recommendations, but their recommendations had to appear to be initiated by the physician.
>
> (Stein, et al., 1990)

In twenty-five years the situation appears to have changed very little.

The bio-medical model tends to be dismissive of caring generally. 'How many nurses fit on top of a scalpel blade?' This is the hidden message of medicine's version of hospital nursing expressed in blatant economic terms. In other words, medical self-interest wants to know how many specialist nurses are needed to enhance *its* specialist medical skills. This instrumental approach is reflected in the current enterprise or cost-effective model in health organisation which sets itself the task of providing a service at a low cost. For instance, if specialist nurses of the future are going to be expensive to educate and retain, then the fewer the better! However, if personalised caring provides a higher quality service enabling patients to recover more quickly, thus using less of the organisation's expensive resources, then nurses may find themselves practising holistic care without a rise in status, job satisfaction, or reward.

Nurses are not angels, they are people caught up within the flow of life in health institutions. As health workers with a relatively low status they have to swim against currents and tides set by various deities who have more power and 'insider' knowledge. Unlike more privileged occupations and groups who make the rules, nurses have to abide by them. The iron rule of obedience in nursing and its required response of deference to *any* authority is not the tail-end of a long line of dominant matrons. It is a consequence of nurses' social or institutional roles as service workers in the hierarchy of health occupations and treatments. What system are nurses being inducted into?

Classified openly as low grade professionals, nurses, especially untrained staff, have an ambiguous status as an intermediary occupation within the organisation. They are neither independent professionals with power, nor mindless manual workers who can be dismissed as purely replaceable labour. On the one hand, their work as the majority of carers is essential to the delivery of a health service which is not totally impersonal. But at the level of health provision where important decisions are taken, their occupational role in caring is marginalised compared as it is to technical and managerial expertise. How can caring be an integral part of medical treatment and yet be so differently rewarded in terms of its occupational expression in low status nursing? This status dilemma is reflected in the views of nursing's leadership. While professional associations encourage patient advocacy, there is an awareness that nurses do not have the structural autonomy over their practices to carry this through.

We know nurses are charged with the responsibility to carry out the orders of others without the authority to affect major decisions concerning approaches to care. This means that nurses do not have the legitimate power in health organisation to initiate caring actions. They do not, therefore, carry out caring as they might choose themselves. Even though nurses now have a right to a professional education, their status in health generally has not radically altered. The change in nurse education is as much a push from nurses themselves as a pull from educational establishments seeking new markets in the vocational area.

Professional education means gaining proficiency and confidence in handling new situations. The majority of nurses however, continue to follow a vocational programme where the emphasis is on practical problem-solving. They learn how to tackle everything except a new situation. Meanwhile, in the practice setting, they do not have the power to affect the framework in which the rules are located. While nurses are seeking a more academic basis to their learning, government policy proposes sending teachers and social workers back to an on-the-spot training. What will be the model for development in the semi-professions? What the State has raised. it can cast aside.

The odd couple: medicine and bureaucracy

In health organisation, nurses' personalised caring has unacknowledged uses in the maintenance of an impersonal system of health care. Someone has to do this because patients are not mindless body parts, and the health service as a human institution does not work like clockwork or by the book. Nurses are not the self-appointed guardians of the patient's self-esteem (measured academically as the patient's right to health). This responsibility is a consequence of their subordinate place as face-to-face carers in a public service institution.

Nurses occupy a particularly interesting position in the provision of health care. Often they are the sole intermediary between the doctor and the patient. At the same time the nurse acts as the buffer between the patient and the potentially bureaucratic nature of the health service.

(Mackay, 1989; p. 4)

As a result: 'the nurse feels she has to be all things to all men and she occasionally gets her responses to expected behaviour mixed.' (Chapman, 1976; p. 113). Doctors need clever pairs of hands to assist them in their technical tasks. Hospital administrators need well-regimented pairs of feet which respond in uniform ways to different marching orders and constant changes in the battle plans. Patients need human compassion, carers who respect them as persons and not merely as bodies. All these groups want what money in a money economy does not necessarily buy. They want the *love* of worker bees, with their dedication of purpose, superb instincts and organisational skills. Who tries to live up to these almost impossibly high and unstated expectations in human caring and who therefore suffers the personal consequences of failing to meet all these needs? Usually nurses in health and usually women in the family and society generally.

Doctors treat patients in the moral-free, objective ways of science and technology. They have a high status as scientific workers. Nurses have a low status because caring, compared as it is to medicine, is seen to be non-scientific and non-technical work. Nursing care in health is regarded as essentially *patient care*. It is low status because it is not seen to have a benefit independent of those who share proprietorship of the patient.

While one elite group (medicine) defines and treats the sick, the other (administration) organises them into the patient role so that the classic medical process can begin. Both have legal and ethical responsibilities to patients as citizens in the provision of a medical service which is safe and healthy. Nurses come somewhere near the bottom line of this professional, institutional responsibility. This means they are in the unacknowledged *front line* of the action. As such they are vulnerable. They have to carry out medical and administrative directives to the letter because the consequences for the doctor or the Health Authority could be dire. Nurses' ethical responsibilities are not directly accountable to the patient but to medical and health authorities. Nurses therefore, have divided loyalties.

The role of nurses involves face-to-face contact with patients. They touch patients, unlike many technical experts who use devices or scanning machines. They can identify patients personally and not only by medical label or a hospital number. Their role is essential in monitoring the effects of various technical and medical treatments on individual patients, particularly in chemotherapy. Nurses' caring roles, however, continue to be defined solely in terms of a manifest utility to the two great powers in health and not in relation to the patient's right to health. Thus the status of nurses and their caring remains dependent upon both medicine and bureaucracy. Nurses are subject to dual institutional roles. One minute they are called upon to do the tidying-up and the next to carry out a real nursing procedure as a part of medical treatment. They must be impersonal routine carers, as well as expert observers of any changes or idiosyncracies in a patient's physical or mental condition.

Medical power exerts control over nurses' behaviour while bureaucracy imposes a different set of rules and controlling standards. Medicine requires careful observation and precision from nurses in carrying out its treatment prescriptions. Bureaucracy in the guise of different styles of management calls for strict obedience to work schedules and supervisory procedures. These codes of conduct expect a degree of flexibility from nursing staff which is not the level openly acknowledged. Junior nurses may be called upon to carry out procedures they have not been formally taught, while senior staff find themselves doing routine physical caring. Nurses as general carers have to extend their official work remit to cover, unofficially, for the work left by someone else.

Health institutions as social institutions lay claim not only to the bodies of nurses and patients but also to their minds. Doctors as the top professionals in health have authority over the mind or mentality of caring. They control entry and all approaches to patient care and treatments. Bureaucracy controls patient behaviour in order to exclude, as much as possible, feelings, emotions, and other messy human affairs from the clinical environment. It has the authority to manage the patient population as well as the body of workers in health care. While medicine requires time and space to carry out its investigations, bureaucracy's over-riding principle of expediency demands that the work be completed as quickly as possible. Patients must be processed in the shortest time to save expensive resources. This is known in nursing as throughput and in sociology as factory or industrial logic.

These versions of patient care present confusing orders for nurses 'at the rockface'. Can nurses conform to both medical and management expectations of conformity? They must act as both the personal servants of administrators and the personal assistants of doctors or other para-medical groups. They are subject to interacting systems of expectations which produce a climate of uncertainty, feelings of personal inadequacy and ambiguity in their authority to act in different situations. Nurses are subject to organisational double standards which are by no means consistently applied.

The valuing of nurses' institutional roles in health is related to the low value of caring in the market place. Caring is not seen to be an acquired skill or even an art but the outcome of a biological destiny. Taken to be essentially women's work, nurses are assumed to be naturally responsible and responsive to people. Nursing care viewed conveniently, as an extension of women's roles in the family serves to conceal that much of this work is hard and dirty. Indeed, some nurses do not think men have the stamina for the job. 'Most of the men I know would not be able to cope with blood, incontinence, diarrhoea – they would be sick and run off to the toilet.' They certainly do not have the inclination! 'It doesn't appeal to men really – cleaning up after people' (Enrolled Nurses, quoted in Mackay, 1989; p. 39). This linking of nurses' roles with womanly virtues, also justifies nurses and their caring as low status. This is not however, the outcome of their intrinsic qualities or a natural logic; it is social prejudice or stereotyping. Nurses have to contend with society's double standards or the unacceptable valuing of people on the basis of their personal attributes rather than hard-earned achievements.

Double burdens: stereotyping of nurses' roles in work and society

Social institutions, whether the family, education, or health, use double standards or inconsistencies in the way they value people. A double standard is the use of different criteria to measure the same or similar behaviour. This is commonly expressed in the saying 'there is one rule for the rich and another for the poor', as well as in the simple but denigrating statement, 'women's work'! People are not solely judged by their achievements but personally, because they are working class *or* female *or* have black skin *or* are too young or too old. Similarly, being poor is often regarded as a personality or behavioural disorder, a lack of assertiveness or competitive drive rather than an objective social condition.

Sociologists take all these labels for what they are – *stereotyping*. This means labelling people as *natural* outsiders because they are *naturally* compliant, *naturally* cunning or just stupid. This is known as the common sense or 'them and us' view. It is used to justify all manner of differences between groups of people as their own fault rather than a serious problem related to some form of social inequity. If these social divisions can be swept under the carpet, that is, relegated to the hidden agenda, then oppressed groups do not have a formal way to express their needs. What is not openly stated as important in needs' hierarchies, whether to do with nurses' attachment to their work or patients' motivation to get well, can be too easily denied. In nursing, the handmaiden's complaints have been taken, historically, to be personal grievances and not problems in service provision. Stress may be a recognised 'fact of life' in nursing, but it is frequently taken to be a personal failing of 'those unable to cope'. Mackay's research (1989) challenges this view.

> Staff shortages and their effects emerged as being the single most important cause of stress. The responsibility for patients' wellbeing can be onerous.
>
> (Mackay, 1989; p. 65)

It is stressful and onerous because the level of responsibility is not openly acknowledged.

Double standards are usually the outcome of deeply held social prejudices (Bauman, 1990). Equal opportunity legislation, for example, is the use of legal means to put the unofficial needs of lower status groups on to open social agendas. These needs are not necessarily hidden, but they are not interpreted as being important compared to those groups who have established a priority. For example, nursing may be a female-intensive occupation but its employing authorities have not taken the needs of women, especially those with family responsibilities, into consideration. Health employers in the past have shown a singular lack of imagination in not providing and integrating part-time work or job-sharing for qualified staff into an actual career structure. Neither have nurses been credited for their organisational abilities in caring for large groups of distressed patients. Administrative prowess is a skill normally associated with male business acumen and not womanly virtues.

Sex-role differences are applied to the evaluation of all types of behaviour. This is shown dramatically in the following verse which appeared originally on a feminist poster.

> A business man is aggressive: a business woman is pushy.
> A business man is good on details: she's picky.
> He loses his temper because he's so involved with his job: she's bitchy.
> He follows through: she doesn't know when to quit.
> He stands firm: she's hard.
> His judgements are her prejudices.
> He is a man of the world: she's been around.
> He drinks because of the excess job pressures: she's a lush.
> He isn't afraid to say what he thinks: she's mouthy.
> He exercises authority diligently: she's power-mad.
> He's close-mouthed: she's secretive.
> He climbed the ladder of success: she's slept her way to the top.
> He's a stern task master: she's hard to work for.
>
> (Source unknown. Quoted in Eichler, 1980; 15)

Mother Theresa, a person respected throughout the world, may be the epitome of womanly virtues but she is also a phenomenal 'tough' organiser! This woman managed to get the needs of the destitute and the dying on to the international health agenda.

It has never been enough for nurses to be brave, to be compassionate, to have the strength to carry on. In nursing these strengths of character have been denigrated as womanly values or vocation, related to a feeling for wanting to work with people. Since feelings are not formally recognised in the world of work these meanings that many nurses may bring to their caring are not recognised or paid for. By way of contrast, similar traits in the elite professions have a high moral value being rewarded in terms of prestige and privilege. The assumptions which inform this differential evaluation of occupational groups are located in a class-bound society. While elite professionals are rewarded for being good people, exercising self-discipline (after all they could just be busy making money), those with a lesser status are seen to be carers out of mere necessity, suggesting a type of determinism rather than conscious moral choice.

Organisational incentives to promote loyalty within high status groups are usually more authority invested, accompanied by an increase in material rewards. Those judged to be of lesser value are urged to work harder! Incentives in nursing tend to take the form of increased regulation or discipline and exhortations to moral duty. Furthermore, it is a hidden management view that below a certain level of status and salary, there are less important work groups whose loyalty will be questionable and therefore require constant supervision. Unfortunately, trainee nurses have been treated as one of these groups; as transitory and disposable labour. Small wonder that many of these young women leave nursing soon after completing their apprenticeship training.

Some occupational groups such as consultants are able to express their needs creatively, making the rules or rising above them. More humble groups cannot exercise such personal judgement in their work, but must be content with satisfying basic physical needs such as earning a living. This division between creative expression and routine work is treated in sociology as a social or class division; measured within the occupational hierarchy as the difference between middle-class and working-class jobs, men's and women's work or intellectual and manual labour.

Needs' hierarchies, which form the basis of organisational agendas, that is, resourcing, allocation, and delegation of tasks, are not immune from the prejudices manifest in the wider society. Thus, well known needs' theorists such as Bloom (1956), Maslow (1970) and Freud (1969), tend to ignore these social divisions in their models depicting the rise from physical to purely intellectual motivators in human behaviour.

Occupational socialisation or learning on the job requires employees to identify with the necessary work tasks and the desired quality of the product. For those in vocational occupations this is a concern to do it to one's own level of satisfaction. This social learning also involves knowing your place or the status mentality which goes with the job relating to its location in the hierarchy as valued highly, lowly, or hardly at all. Those in authority positions must learn to curb their privileges. They have the moral task of pursuing the status attached to their positions but not to resort to using this power for personal reasons. Nurses, and other less powerful groups, also have difficult moral tasks but these stem from relative deprivation not privilege. They must acquire a generalised deference to any authority. This is not something which human beings take to very lightly. It usually requires open military-style discipline or an efficient hidden agenda to enforce it.

Nurses' social roles are the outcome of a health system which has covertly relied upon their work as highly skilled generalists to clean up the mess other health workers leave behind. Having shown that they can do this very professionally, many nurses assume that it means promotion. But professional status or privilege is not necessarily conferred from above purely on the grounds of merit; nor is it necessarily desirable. In occupational sociology, professionalism replaces class as the prevailing system of dominance or supremacy. The place of nurses in health professionalism is the outcome of an industrial or technical division of labour compounded by the problem of gender.

> Of all the professions subject to sex-role stereotyping, nursing seems the most severely handicapped in that nurses are doubly conditioned into playing a subservient role: first by society generally, and secondly, by the medical establishment.
>
> (Pizurki, et al., quoted in Robinson, J., 1989; p. 163)

The low status and rewards of women's work are not only due to the type of work they do, but their lower social status as domestic marginal beings. Their need for support is supposed to reside in the family, not work. Gender is not the only explanation of nursing's place in health; but it is the only socially acceptable one. Female-intensive occupations are often seen as ritualistic, rule-governed, context-bound and lacking autonomy. Gender, or more explicitly 'femaleness', used as an explanatory variable is taken to be 'backwardness'. Low morale, a much discussed problem in health, is associated with low efficiency. Low pay and low status lead to low morale. What stands in the way of low morale in nursing? More men in nursing has not raised its status or morale, only increased the competition for senior posts. More specialist posts mean higher pay for the few, but may cause the status of the majority of nurses and helper groups to decline (Salvage, 1985).

In sociology nursing has been referred to as a 'semi' *or* feminine *or* caring *or* welfare profession (Abbott and Wallace, 1990b). But a more realistic term would be under-profession. For nursing has truly been overshadowed by both medical and government definitions of its interests and the direction of its practices. It has been prescribed primarily in terms of a *work ethic*; as physical care and instrumental tasks. This is a purely management definition whereby nurses are the instruments of organisational work prescriptions.

Sociological explanations of nursing take into account the interaction of economic class and enduring notions of femininity. Nurses have been a source of cheap labour; constituting their economic function. At the same time their socialization has been explictly gendered in that they carry out emotional and unpaid work. Both are servicing roles. Nurses constitute a servant or lower class within the professional hierarchy. While their unpaid vocation is emphasised, even publicised, as the human face of a largely technical system, it is also used to justify a lack of overall commitment to more meaningful concepts of care or increased status for carers. In nursing, where the professional ideology does not correspond to the reality, the higher the altruism expected the stronger the justification for lower prestige and rewards.

Sociological accounts of nursing start from an understanding of its complex role in health and welfare institutions. Openly, nurses have to ensure that bureaucratic objectives are achieved and that the tasks of patient care are accomplished. Covertly, nurses socialise patients into the passive sick role so that the doctor-patient relationship can take place. Their domestic involvement with patients and their families is an unacknowledged part of wider welfare structures which support people in times of need. In obvious economic terms, nurses make up the largest single group of carers in the health industry. Covertly, they have been used like an endless supply of cheap and replaceable labour. Nurses have caring as well as custodial roles; nursing has open as well as hidden functions. These manifold functions are summarised below.

Social functions of Nursing: care and custody, open and hidden.

1. *Social caring*:
   - caring as routine, physical activity; housework, hygiene and technical tasks;
   - nurturing of patients to encourage independence, known in nursing as personalised caring.
2. *Social control*:
   - instrumental role offers protection of the person from the harsh realities of people's suffering;

- nurses encourage patient passivity so that the medical process can take place;
- nurses socialise and supervise other nurses into compliance within the health service culture.

3. *Social meanings or ideology*:
   - professional ideology of patient advocacy
   - different approaches to work, for example vocational or work ethic (just a job);
   - ethical responsibilities derived from the needs of higher authorities, not the patients.

4. *Economic uses*:
   - central role as direct producers of care;
   - used as generalists to uphold technical specialism;
   - source of cheap labour (throughput was applied to nurses prior to its application in processing patients).

5. *Political implications*:
   - supports the struggle over patients' rights in health care;
   - nurses do not have the power to decide how caring takes place because others do;
   - in terms of power, nursing can be compared almost to that of a minority group, especially those who work in the community.

Generations of nurses have not been born to the job, instead they have been moulded in definite ways. All manner of ritualistic practices, outmoded beliefs, accusations of compliance or non-assertiveness, and the self-deprecatory feelings that nurses project on to each other and nursing as a whole, can be attributed conveniently to nurses themselves because they are part of a mainly female and practical occupation. These are not personality characteristics but organisational problems. Distinctions between medicine and nursing, cure and care, are not natural extensions of male, technical expertise or female passivity but social divisions. If we abolish socially acceptable distinctions between medicine and nursing, on the grounds that these are neither natural nor essential divisions, what do we get?

The unquiet marriage: care and cure

Who are the 'natural' winners?

Sociology studies the way society values people. Modes of valuing people whether based upon science, technological expertise, religion or magic are not timeless truths but social judgements. Sociologists assume that no distinction between individuals or groups expressed in terms of differential power, prestige and rewards are purely natural, even when there are obvious biological differences such as gender, age, or race. Status distinctions between social activities associated with what men or women do are not natural but cultural products. They are the product of social divisions or inequalities which over time become acceptable as the natural order of things. All this means is that a certain form of social supremacy, masquerading as 'tradition', has been carrying on unquestioned for some time; creating and establishing dependency among all those not accepted into its elite province. Control and dependency are two intimately connected features of any couple relationship within unequal class and gendered societies; whether between doctor and patient, doctor and nurse, employer and employee or husband and wife. What counts in this system? More importantly, what is discounted?

Who is seen to be stupid?

There is no natural distinction between care and cure, nursing and medicine. These differences are the products of history and definite social practices, not logic. Superior social status does not necessarily mean superior expertise in solving particular human problems. Similarly, a lack of superior status does not mean that people are worthless, only worth less compared with the skills and outlook of more powerful groups.

In a middle-class society, middle-class jobs are associated with intellectual content and creative expression while manual work, no matter how creative or useful to society, may be classified as almost mindless. Since work identity is closely linked to personal identity and vice versa, people frequently underestimate the awareness and intelligence of those with a lesser status. Doctors may be openly admiring of clever doctors but they do not apply the same values to clever nurses (Mackay, 1989).

Why are the majority of carers women?

Caring may be an integral part of medical cure and every person's health and sanity but in the present system it is devalued as either women's work or something that good people do naturally, meaning **unthinkingly**. Learning to care tends to be viewed as a personality attribute, passively acquired during general socialisation. It is not supposed to require formal learning, thus denying the demands that are made on people as they adjust to their caring roles 'on the job'. In the past nurses' educational programmes heavily endorsed character-building or moral worthiness. The stress was on learning the rules of middle-class behaviour and putting the needs of others before your own. This moral socialisation remains a large part of nurses' vocational education today – the unacknowledged part.

The study of professionalism in sociology is not about altruism but power and occupation. Health professionalism, immersed within scientific education, undervalues social caring and knowledge gained from direct experience. When nurses carry out caring they do so within social medical institutions. They come up against higher authorities who can use scientific justifications to explain the supremacy of their versions of how nurses should approach and care for patients. The views of trainee nurses or patients, their self-definitions of need, confront not just doctors or managers but the whole scientific (predominantly male) establishment. It is hardly surprising that many nurses may experience feelings of intimidation, fear and even shame.

Sociologists take these feelings of personal inadequacy seriously and attempt to explain them as organisational dilemmas. All the classic sociologists, Marx, Weber and Durkheim, addressed themselves to the problem of alienation, or the disenchantment with work in the twentieth century. Alienation is the separation of the mentality and execution of tasks according to social and occupational divisions (Braverman, 1974; Storch and Stinson, 1988).

> It may be argued that nurses in the NHS have always been subject to bureaucratic control and that nursing has therefore always been proletarian by nature . . . the progressive fragmentation of work leads to a situation where knowledge about the whole task is separated from the execution of its component parts. Indeed, the tasks may be allocated to different groups of workers outside the control of nursing
>
> (Robinson, J., 1991; p. 295)

As stated earlier, nurses do not control the mentality of caring because others do. The intelligence and interest needed to carry out their work willingly, is appropriated by two principal entities, medicine and management. Nurses do not carry out caring as they might choose themselves.

Why are most professionals men?

The problem is not one of too many passive and unambitious women. The answer is that gender is mainly class disposition and inheritance. For instance, medicine in England is an elite profession, considered to be an appropriate career mainly for men from established, upper middle-class backgrounds. If this type of work was randomly selected on the basis of individual inclination or talent then the class, gender, age and ethnic composition of medicine would be somewhat different. One would expect a random distribution of specific social groups, similar to their presence in the population generally. In the same vein, if doctors pursued their public service ethic, that is, patient need and not technical specialism, then the majority would be gerontologists, psychiatrists or spiritual healers. Despite the views of many doctors, medicine continues to place surgery and transplant surgery above all other specialisms. Meanwhile, the majority of patients suffer from chronic, rather than acute illnesses which require long-term management and care. Technological medicine is wonderful if the patient is carried in on a stretcher. It is not, however, very useful for the many walking around with numerous debilitating conditions.

Why are most doctors in Russia women?

Comparative study of health systems reveals that the same jobs may be associated with different genders. In Russia until recently over 95 per cent of physicians were female (Navarro, 1977). It appears that women are not naturally best suited to be nurses, nor men to be doctors. The reason for the overwhelming female presence in Russian medicine, and for the feminised nature of British nursing, is that the work is of relatively low status in the professional hierarchy. In both examples, the work these women do is controlled and overseen by a 'top heavy', state bureaucracy. Consequently, their roles are primarily regulated by institutional rules and not a professional self-discipline. The issue here may be more to do with external authority than gender.

In the British system as in the former Soviet model, bureaucracy increasingly sets itself up as the sole arbiter of standards in health. Caring expertise, separated from a professional basis in particular groups, becomes a centralised function of management, the 'Great Leveller'. Science and artistic standards come together, supposedly, in an impersonal bureaucracy expressed in various styles of modern management. While this raises the professional status of administrators and managers, enhancing their careers, it tends to down-grade everyone else, including doctors.

Why are many nurse managers men?

Nurses who become managers are managers first and foremost. Their definitions of nursing problems and solutions arise out of organisational needs rather than preoccupation with nursing interventions in the patient's right to health. In this context, male nurses are seen to be more capable of socially distancing themselves from the needs of (1) direct practitioners who are, after all, mainly female and (2) the majority of patients who are also predominantly female (especially in the very elderly group). 'More men are entering nursing and new managerial structures introduced in the 1970s have resulted in a disproportionately large number of men appointed to management posts' (Abbott and Wallace, 1990a; p. 24).

The hidden message here may be that male managers are perceived by their superiors, also mainly men though of a higher social class, as capable of taking moral-free decisions. In other words, that they are more likely to base decisions on financial resources (the money) and not enter debates about whose needs are not being met (the quality of provision). This degrades the contribution of not only female but also caring male nurses. However, the high proportion of men in nurse management does serve to maintain the gap between direct producers and consumers of care in terms of a status of gender, as well as occupational position. If this trend continues, divisions within nursing between those who do the caring and those who supervise it, intensify and widen.

Why is caring taken to be menial work?

The particular quality which gives medicine supremacy in health is its covert power based upon a combination of class and male dominance. Nursing has achieved a certain middle-class respectability, but its status is not defined independent of its use to medicine and administration. Nurses continue to have a lower middle-class propriety, a correctness of behaviour or character, which does not threaten the medical ownership of the patient as private property. Within the framework of the health service, nursing becomes almost a working-class or manual job. In relation to market forces, this implies that nurses are general not expert labour, and they have been used and paid accordingly. Nursing care, labelled as essentially practical activity by those who have the power to conceptualise its tasks, is low status in a system which values technical experts, including administrators, above all others. Caring is an essential part of any person's experience of illness *or* dying *or* recovery *or* well-being. However, caring in industrial society and in health has a low market value. Secretaries are industry's handmaidens in the commercial arena; nurses have been the equivalent in the health sector.

The social control of nursing and caring by higher status occupations means it continues to be regulated in terms of commonplace tasks which specialists apparently cannot be bothered with themselves. This is the nurses' role within the social order in health. They also contribute to the patient's self-esteem. Their roles emerge from an enormous clash of social values between instrumental models of care and personalised caring; between *social control* of patients' and nurses' behaviour and *human values* based upon experience and self-definitions of need. The under-valuing of nurses in health is linked to the de-valuing of carers, producers, the family, and spirituality in consumer societies.

Nurses have an intense personal responsibility for patients which contrasts vividly with the impersonal approaches of medicine and bureaucracy. Administrators and doctors have the authoritative task of taking moral-free decisions between groups competing for their resources, thereby relinquishing carers who may be biased, from the need to make decisions. This is the rhetoric but what is the reality? Nursing care, imbued as it is with human meaning, relieves these technical experts of a considerable responsibility for patients' personal needs. How important this quality is to a patient's recovery we do not know as it is vastly under-researched. We do know that this work is central to the continued running of the health service and the maintenance of the doctor-patient relationship. Along with other direct producers, nursing care is part of the huge amount of activity which has to happen before the classic, medical process can begin and top administrators 'turn up' for work.

Can medicine solve society's health problems?

In popular imagery, nursing is seen to be a health profession closely associated with the work doctors do. At times, doctors and nurses do work side-by-side, but the social distance between these occupations, measured in terms of class, status and power, is considerable. Medicine takes its established place in health for granted. Even though its definition is narrow, its social power over populations is widespread. Alone medicine cannot solve society's health problems, but it is taken to be the model for all developments in health, and an indicator of professional status throughout society.

Nursing, viewed as a deviation from the medical model taken to be the norm, is found to be wanting in numerous ways. Though nurses question this social power to define patient's needs and roles, they rarely ask what it means in terms of definitions of their own roles. If treatment for the sick is subject to bureaucratic rules and professional control, then caring for the sick is stratified and diversified. Thus the ranking order in nursing is the product of the social hierarchy of specialisms in clinical categories as well as occupations.

> types of nursing that are valued are determined by the priorities set by the biomedical model . . . Nursing in a geriatric unit, in a long-stay psychiatric hospital, in district nursing and in other non-cure areas was regarded with lower esteem, and these areas were thought of as the places where the less-bright nurse who could not cope or had blotted her copy-book ended up.
>
> (Pearson and Vaughan, 1986; pp. 22–3)

All professional relationships in health are mediated through medical categories which means the minds, experience, and the behaviour of doctors, and increasingly, state administrators. It is their need for status and independence, not nurse or patient need, which determines health organisation.

Who are the professionals dependent upon?

There is considerable discussion in nursing theory on the status and psychological dependency of patients within the bio-medical model. There is very little discussion on the status and psychological dependency of professionals on patients. For example, professional nursing models encourage contradictory tasks; on the one hand patient advocacy which assumes a patient's right to define their health, and on the other professionalism which presupposes patient dependency. The patient role is vital to an understanding of the professional role of the nurse or the doctor (Davies, 1979).

It may seem obvious to state that doctors and administrators have a high status and nurses and patients do not. Patient and nurse passivity is not a natural response to superior expertise, it is an acquired deference to authority. An essential part of the socialization of nurses or patients is the learning of a low status mentality which equates with their imposed, institutional roles. This is one of the main sources of discontent in nursing which nurses project on to each other. The maintenance of control in any field is largely dependent upon subordinate groups identifying with the needs of authority figures to the detriment of their own needs. The way this effect is achieved in health care and other social institutions may take the form of informal or unstated processes involving persuasion or even coercion. This social learning is called, as we have seen, the hidden agenda.

Pyramids of power: the nursing context

An underlying theme throughout this discussion has been constructed powerlessness in nursing. This contrasts with prevailing views of nursing as either an independent profession, or a naturally passive female workforce. I have attempted to show that the primary responsibility of nurses is not to nursing values but the organisations in which they work. For it is a basic tenet in sociology, that workers are not only educated and trained to perform certain tasks but to reproduce a defined, formal way of doing things which militates against change. Thus nurses enter nursing because they like to 'work with people', but along the way they find that the intentions of their work are usually for the benefit of higher authorities and not the patient. This has lead nurses to question health service priorities and the handmaiden mentality:

> It has to make sense to put the patient's rather than the doctor's interests first. How can we say we are delivering patient-centred care when the likes and dislikes of doctors determine our care? . . . the nurse's role must be defined within a system that doesn't have medical knowledge at its pinnacle.
>
> (Jones, 1987; p. 59)

Despite all the seeming diversity in the present health industry, the structure remains bureaucratic or hierarchical. Hierarchies of need are still grounded in the bio-medical or hospital model of illness, while access to treatments via the 'free' Health Service is more difficult to attain. This concentration of power at the top of the pyramid, explains the stability over time of inequalities in authority and rewards, and in particular, the continuing subordinate status of nurses tied as they are to medical and managerial versions of caring.

> A true patient-centred model for nursing practice, which imbues the client with power over decision-making, would be a direct challenge to the tightly controlled boundaries . . . between the roles of the doctor [and] the nurse . . . it is unlikely that such a model for practice would be welcomed by those whose power it seeks to remove.
>
> (Keyzer, 1988; p. 105)

Power is not always associated with dominance and submission, as in the spiritual power to heal, to nurture or to self-care. Similarly, discipline is not necessarily chastisement or punishment resulting in compliance. It is a code of moral conduct or creed to enable an individual to live according to collective rules, faith and self-government. Chastisement only comes into this interaction if the rules are broken. Discipline and power supposedly come together in professional practice where public service and the promotion of independence in others takes precedence over self-interest. For instance, lay people define a professional as a good person, someone who can be appealed to in times of need; who does not take advantage of people when they are truly vulnerable. This ideal version of the professional role may not coincide with the reality of many practitioners, be they doctors or nurses.

Professional ideology is not the only explanation of practice and it may be misleading. Increasingly, all professional roles are defined within large-scale organisations in which the individual's 'keeping of the faith' is overwhelmed by management prescriptions of accountability and loyalty to 'The Firm': 'The result is that professionals have become subordinate employees within the control of centralised bureaucracies' (Robinson, J 1991; p. 295)

Nowadays we may know who is in charge but not who is morally responsible for standards. In the money/quality debate that rages in the Health Service which side are nurses on?

The new managerialism in nursing (Carpenter, 1977) does not mean that nurses have more say as well as more responsibility in the way they carry out caring. In the context of the current nursing hierarchy, management acts as a mechanism of increasing control over nurses' work. This may result in a further lack of morale and suppression of the freedom to question practices. The change from a military to an industrial hierarchy has not alleviated the intense discipline and climate of intimidation. The majority of nurses are still regarded as pairs of hand or feet whether they are supervising manual tasks or actually doing them. The importance of physical care in patient recovery, carried out mainly by trainees and helpers, continues to be held in low social esteem. Nurses need to redefine their roles not just in nursing service or education but in terms of wider health organisation.

Order and disorder: the summary

Once upon a time in the health service, doctors consulted, bureaucrats administered resources, nurses had ethical responsibilities and patients had a right to treatment, free at the point of access. This is the beginning of the official story of healthcare as a purely public-spirited service. The reality, however, is not located in an assumed consensus but occupational and individual conflicts. Health workers are members of *different social classes* who are affected by status distinctions at work. Those in middle management (the level to which nurse managers may rise) have the impossible task of trying to hold all these disparate groups together.

Until the 1970s the structure of the health service resembled a fairly closed feudal order with fixed boundaries between skill and authority. Consultants had power like lords in their manors, bureaucrats gained control of the treasury and ruled like barons, nurses had to obey orders without question like bonded servants, and patients or the peasantry had to accept any scientific truth as long as it was not their own.

In the current model, the industrial system has taken hold. The class of barons or bureaucrats have gained control not only over resources but the whole organisation. The health service under government direction means many health workers have to live up to an enterprise ideal in which the principle of expediency is used to justify any means to obtain the result of 'throughput'. Science and artistic standards have been separated from a traditional basis in professional or vocational groups and now come together in an administrative lay elite.

Consultants, as private practitioners, may have their own practices to go to. The majority of doctors, as general practitioners, are accountable to a definite budget, patient quotas and an enormous amount of time-consuming paper work. Some nurses may have access to managerial careers but this has not led to increased nursing control over the mentality or content of caring. Patients have consumer rights to select treatments between competing hospitals, but without access to the knowledge which they need to make informed choices. Many individual health workers may find it difficult to live down to the impersonal logic of a factory production line in processing patients as quickly as possible. But most importantly for our analysis here is that

> one consistent and key factor has emerged from the findings of the Nursing Policy Studies Centre's . . . empirical research into the management of nursing after Griffiths . . . that is the invisibility of most nursing issues to everyone except nurses.
>
> (Robinson, 1989; p. 154)

The invisibility of nursing issues is not, as we have seen, the fault of nurses but their social location in health.

Sociology, unlike the natural sciences, is not primarily concerned with presenting new discoveries. Instead it teaches new ways of looking at things with which we are familiar. In this chapter I have raised and discussed many old problems in nursing, relating these to nurses' concealed, extensive use in health organisation. For the handmaiden role has been an historic prerequisite to the evaluation of classic, hospital medicine and administration.

I have attempted to show that:

1. Nurses are socialised into 'knowing their place' through the sheer weight of social institutions and prevailing definitions of Science (Robinson, 1991; p. 299).
2. The social institution of medicine is not just doctors.

In health professionalism, nursing care has been taken to be non-scientific patient care; a derivative of medicine and management. Caring has not been seen in a meaningful way, independent of curative science or technical expertise. Nurses' social roles emerge from the manufacture of an industrial system of health rather than a professional ethos: 'The curative model . . . borrowed not from gender relations in the wider society but from the organisation of the factory' (Bellaby and Oribabor, 1980; p. 163). The key to understanding what nursing is when it happens lies not in openly stated health intentions, but within the hidden agenda where tensions resulting from unequal exchanges between occupations and work groups are relegated and evaded. Nurses' roles are openly defined in instrumental ways, their personalised caring tending to come into informal health practices – the hidden agenda. While great strides have been made recently to develop a new official curriculum in nurse education, the impact of the hidden agenda has not been explored in depth.

When I started to write this chapter I was puzzled by the question: How does the complexity of nursing care become reduced to its context-bound place in the health order? But the questions I have tried to answer here, using sociology, are more specific. Who is defining it as unimportant in the first place, and who benefits? For hidden agendas are primarily concerned with ensuring that some are set up to fail, while the destined winners succeed. This is an enduring feature of health care in class and gender-structured societies. If the health order is based upon a hierarchy of inequalities in power and rewards, the authority/compliance divide, then it is unlikely to meet the needs of many groups of people in society today.

References

Adams, A. (1991). *Bullying at Work*. (Radio Four Factsheet) BBC, London.

Abbott, P. and Wallace, C. (1990a). Social work and nursing: a history. In *The Sociology of the Caring Professions*, P. Abbott and C. Wallace (eds), pp. 10–28. Falmer, London.

Abbott, P. and Wallace, C. (eds) (1990b). *The Sociology of the Caring Professions*. Falmer, London.

Bauman, Z. (1990). *Thinking Sociologically*. Basil Blackwell, Oxford.

Bedell, G. (1992). The lazy guide to office success. *The Independent On Sunday*, 8 March, 20.

Becher, T. (1989). *Academic Tribes and Territories*. Open University Press, Milton Keynes.

Bellaby, P. and Oribabor, P. (1980). The history of the present-contradiction and struggle in nursing. In *Rewriting Nursing History*, C. Davies (ed.), pp. 147–74. Croom Helm, London.

Bloom, B.S. (ed.) (1956). *Taxonomy of Learning Objectives*: the Classification of Educational Goals. Handbook 1. Cognitive Domain*. Longman, London.

Braverman, H. (1974). *Labor and Monopoly Capital*: the Degradation of Work in the Twentieth Century*. Monthly Review Press, New York.

Carpenter, M. (1977). The new managerialism and professionalism in nursing. In *Health and the Division of Labour*, M. Stacey, M. Reid, C. Heath and R. Dingwall (eds), pp. 165–93. Croom Helm, London.

Chapman, C. (1976). The use of sociological theories and models in nursing. *Journal of Advanced Nursing*, **1(2)**, 111–27.

Davies, C. (1979). Comparative occupational roles in health care. *Social Science and Medicine*. **13A(5)**, 515–21.

Eichler, M. (1980). *The Double Standard*: a Feminist Critique of Feminist Social Science*. Croom Helm, London.

Faugier, J. (1991). Courage rules OK. *Nursing Times*, **87(23)**, 22.

Freidson, E. (1970). *Profession of Medicine*: a Study of the Sociology of Applied Knowledge*. Dodd, Mead, New York.

Freud, S. (1969). *An Outline of Psycho Analysis*. Hogarth Press, London.

Giddens, A. (1989). *Sociology*. Polity. Cambridge.

Heenan, A. (1990). Playing patients. *Nursing Times*, **86(46)**, 46–8.

Ho, E. (1989). The 'hidden curriculum' in midwifery education. *Midwives Chronicle*, **102**, 291–3.

Howton, F.W. (1969). *Functionaries*. Quadrangle Books, Chicago.

Jolley, M. and Brykczyńska, G. (eds) (1992). *Nursing Care*: the Challenge to Change*. Edward Arnold, London.

Jones, C. (1987). Handmaiden mentality. *Nursing Times*, **83(40)**, 59.

Katzman, E.M. and Roberts, J.I. (1988). Nurse-physician conflicts as barriers to the enactment of nursing roles. *Western Journal of Nursing Research*, **10(5)**, 576–90.

Keddy, B., Gillis, M.J., Jacobs, P., Burton, H. and Rogers, M. (1986). The doctor-nurse relationship: an historical perspective. *Journal of Advanced Nursing*, **11(6)**, 745–53.

Keyzer, D.M. (1988). Challenging role boundaries: conceptual frameworks for understanding the conflict arising from the implementation of the nursing process in practice. In *Political Issues in Nursing*: *Past*, *Present and Future*. *Volume* 3. R. White (ed.), pp. 95–119. Wiley, Chichester.

Mackay, L. (1989). *Nursing a Problem*. Open University Press, Milton Keynes.

Mackay, L. (1990). Nursing: just another job? In *The Sociology of the Caring Professions*, P. Abbott and C. Wallace (eds), pp. 29–39. Falmer, London.

Maslow, A. (1970). *Motivation and Personality*, 2nd ed. Harper & Row, New York.

Melia, K.M. (1984). Student nurses' construction of occupational socialisation. *Sociology of Health and Illness*, **6(2)**, 132–51.

Melia, K.M. (1987). *Learning and Working*: *the Occupational Socialization of Nurses*. Tavistock, London.

Merton, R. (1973). *The Sociology of Science*. University of Chicago, Chicago.

Navarro, V. (1977). *Social Security and Medicine in the USSR*. Heath, Lexington.

Pearson, A. and Vaughan, B. (1986). *Nursing Models for Practice*. Heinemann, London.

Perry, A. (1991). Sociology-its contributions and critiques. In *Nursing a Knowledge Base for Practice*, A. Perry and M. Jolley (eds), pp. 154–98. Edward Arnold, London.

Roget's Thesaurus of English Words and Phrases (1962). Longman, London.

Robinson, J. (1986). Covering up for the doctor. *Nursing Times*, **82(30)**, 35–6.

Robinson, J. (1989). Nursing in the future: a cause for concern. In *Current Issues in Nursing*, M. Jolley and P. Allan (eds), pp. 151–78. Chapman and Hall, London.

Robinson, J. (1991). Power, politics and policy analysis in nursing. In *Nursing – a Knowledge Base for Practice*. A. Perry and M. Jolley (eds), pp. 271–307. Edward Arnold, London.

Salvage, J. (1985). *The Politics of Nursing*. Heinemann, London.

Savage, W. (1986). *Savage Enquiry*. Virago, London.

Stacey. M., Reid. M., Heath. C. and Dingwall. R. (eds) (1977). *Health and the Division of Labour*. Croom Helm, London.

Stein. L. (1967). The doctor-nurse game. *Archives of General Psychiatry*, **16**, 699–703.

Stein. L.I., Watts. D.T. and Howell. T. (1990). The doctor-nurse game revisited. *The Lamp*, **47(9)**, 23–6.

Stockwell, F. (1972). *The Unpopular Patient*. Royal College of Nursing, London.

Storch, J.L. and Stinson, S.M. (1988). Concepts of deprofessionalization with applications to nursing. In *Political Issues in Nursing*: *Past*, *Present and Future*, *Volume 3*. R. White (ed.), pp. 33–44. Wiley, Chichester.

Strong. P. and Robinson. J. (1988). *New Model Management*: *Griffiths and the NHS*. Nursing Policy Studies Centre. University of Warwick, Conventry.

Turner. T. (1991). A paper tiger? *Nursing Times*, **87(24)**, 20.

White. R. (1988). The influence of nursing on the politics of health. In *Political*

Issues in Nursing: *Past, Present and Future*, *Volume three*, R. White (ed.), pp. 15–31. Wiley, Chichester.

Suggestions for further reading

Adam, A. (1992). *Bullying at work: how to confront and overcome it*. Virago, London.
Albrow, M. (1970). *Bureaucracy*. Macmillan. London.
Bauman, Z. (1989). *Modernity and the Holocaust*. Policy, Cambridge, ch. 6: The Ethics of Obedience: Reading Milgram.
Dolan, N. (1987). The relationship between burnout and job satisfaction in nurses. *Journal of Advanced Nursing*, **12(1)**, 3–12.
Eldridge, J.E.T. and Crombie, A.D. (1974). *A Sociology of Organisations*. Allen & Unwin, London.
Foucault, M. (1980). *Power/Knowledge*: *selected interviews* and *other writings, 1972–1977*. C. Gordon, (ed.). Harvester Press, Brighton.
Gaze, H. (1987). Man appeal. *Nursing Times*, **83(20)**, 24–7.
Hardy, L. (1987). The male model. *Nursing Times*, **83(21)**, 36–8.
Payne, R. and Firth-Sozens, J. (eds) (1987). *Stress in Health Professionals*. Wiley, Chichester.
Robinson, J. (1991). Educational conditioning. *Nursing Times*, **87(10)**, 28–31.
Schaef, A.W. and Fassel, D. (1990). *The Addictive Organisation*. Harper & Row, New York.
White. R. (ed.) (1988). *Political Issues in Nursing: Past, Present and Future*. *Volume 3*. Wiley, Chichester.

4 Hidden curricula in nursing education

> Miss *Jonesy* bent to pick a rose,
> A rose so sweet and slender;
> Alas! Alack! She bent too far
> And bang went her suspender.
> (Opie and Opie, 1959)

Learning to use humour as a way of coping with the demands of school life is something most, if not all, readers will have experienced. For verses about teachers and practical jokes perpetrated upon them help in some measure to redress the power differential between teacher and taught, and humour in general can be used 'to defeat boredom and fear, to overcome hardship and problems – as a way out of almost anything' (Willis, 1977). Such learning does not form part of teacher intentions embodied in the formal curriculum, and for children humour is part of their taken-for-granted school experience. In this sense, then, such learning forms part of a hidden curriculum. The concept of 'hidden curriculum', however, is by no means straightforward. Indeed, as Giroux (1983) points out, 'What are at stake in the divergent styles and modes of analyses that make up the literature on the hidden curriculum are deep-seated philosophical and ideological perspectives that clash over the very meaning and nature of social reality.'

This chapter will begin by discussing some of the relevant terminology used in the literature in order to explore different interpretations of what a hidden curriculum *is*. This will be followed by a review of the sort of learning which can occur via a hidden curriculum: the strategies students may use to 'get by' and the messages they may receive from their school/college environment. The significance of the concept 'hidden curriculum' will be explored in the context of nursing education and suggestions will be made as to how insights drawn from the literature can illuminate practice and help nurse educators facilitate truly educational experiences with their students.

Defining hidden curriculum

Jenkins and Shipman (1976) mention the 'unwritten yet potent set of influences exerted through the organisation of schools and they state that 'The hidden curriculum includes all those pervasive values that one is expected to acquire by a process of institutional seepage: things like punctuality, good behaviour, tolerance of frustration, loyalty.' In this account, although the influences are unwritten, the phrase 'expected to acquire' suggests that there is some *conscious intention* that students do in fact acquire these values. This element of the curriculum could therefore be described as hidden because it is unwritten and possibly because the students are not aware of the process of 'institutional seepage'. A different view is taken by Eggleston (1977), who, discarding the distinction between the official curriculum and the hidden curriculum suggests that 'What we are seeing is in fact two perspectives on the total curriculum – the official curriculum that is predominantly a teacher perspective and the hidden curriculum that is predominantly a student perspective.' The difference between this account and that of Jenkins and Shipman lies in the fact that Eggleston stresses students' active use of strategies to 'get by' in the system and the potential power they have to control the productivity of the classroom (the learning) by, for example, working to rule or bargaining with teachers. Eggleston (1977) however, concludes that 'the hidden curriculum is as one with the official curriculum as an instrument of social control in which students, like teachers, have for the most part only the power to conform'. The notion of social control is reiterated by Vallance (1977) who states that she uses the term hidden curriculum to refer to 'those non-academic but educationally significant consequences of schooling that occur systematically but are not made explicit at any level of the public rationales for education . . . It refers broadly to the social control function of schooling'.

Vallance's (1977) definition is interesting not only because she emphasises social control but also because she attempts to clarify how she interprets 'hidden'. Martin (1976) discusses this aspect of 'hiddenness' at some length. She argues that there are two kinds of hiddenness and both relate to intent. Something like a cure for cancer, she suggests, can be hidden from us in the sense of being unknown to us. On the other hand, a penny hidden in a children's game has been hidden *with intent by someone*. Martin (1976) stresses the importance of clarifying this ambiguity, for if social control exercised via a hidden curriculum is intentional then it does not make sense to try and tinker with school practices in order to do away with a hidden curriculum. In view of the popularity of the hidden curriculum among social scientists Hargreaves (1980) wonders from whom the hidden curriculum is now hidden and he proposes instead the term 'paracurriculum' – that which is taught and learned alongside the formal or official curriculum'. The problem with Hargreaves' (1980) definition, however, is that it fails to allow for the possibility that learning of a non-explicit nature may occur via the content of the official curriculum. A further point about Hargreaves' (1980) analysis is his contention that *the* hidden curriculum has now been unmasked.

This could suggest that there is *one* hidden curriculum which once discovered no longer holds any mysteries. Yet elsewhere Hargreaves recognises that though the *concept* of the hidden curriculum is now well-known, clarification is still needed about, for example, how the contents or 'subjects' vary. This is an issue explored by Martin (1976) who stresses that 'A hidden curriculum, like a curriculum proper, is *of* some setting, *at* some time, and *for* some learner.'

Before concluding this examination of different interpretations of 'hidden curriculum', one or two of the points already discussed will be considered in relation to the nursing literature. Alexander (1982), for example, distinguishes between

> 'theory', defined as the subject matter of nursing as it is taught in the classroom, block, or college of nursing, i.e. the material of the formal or overt curriculum, with 'practice', defined as what is done when the nurse is engaged in giving nursing care in the wards or other clinical areas. The latter is what in present day parlance is termed the 'hidden curriculum' . . . – the curriculum which, in nursing, is a potent force in transmitting the values, the beliefs about the 'way nursing is'.
>
> (Alexander, 1982)

Alexander's interpretation highlights some of the complexity of the concept 'hidden curriculum'. If, for example, students practise unsafely on the wards because they have been taught unsafely by the ward staff, this could be seen as an example of the *actual* curriculum' (Kelly, 1989) not being in accord with official curricular intentions. To take another example, if college teaching is out of touch with the realities of clinical practice, and yet students practise safely and flexibly because they have been well taught by the ward staff, then it could be argued that the *actual* curriculum taught by the teaching staff is unsatisfactory. It could also be that the official curriculum needs updating! On the other hand, strategies used by students to cope with the demands of the organisation such as 'looking busy' (Melia, 1981) are likely to be learnt by 'institutional seepage' rather than direct, intentional teaching from ward staff, and so would seem to be part of the hidden curriculum. Moreover, the way work is organised on wards may transmit tacit messages to students about 'the way nursing is', and this too would appear to be part of a hidden curriculum.

The task of defining a hidden curriculum is made more complicated by the fact that, as Vallance (1977) points out, a number of 'satellite labels' are attached to the concept of hidden curriculum: the 'unstudied curriculum', the 'covert' or 'latent' curriculum, the 'non-academic outcomes of schooling', the 'by-products of schooling', the 'residue of schooling' or just 'what schooling does to people'; (Overly, 1970; Vallance, 1972) (both cited by Vallance, 1977). However, as Meighan (1986) argues, ambiguous notions such as 'hidden curriculum' are valuable because like de Bono's 'porridge words' they can be stirred around to stimulate further ideas and connections. The *danger* of ambiguous words occurs when the meaning slips and slides without warning so that 'attempted analysis is replaced by spurious association' (Meighan, 1986). Kelly (1989) appears to recognise this problem and he discusses 'hidden curriculum' and differentiates between official and actual curricula, and formal and informal curricula, as well as offering a definition of 'curriculum'.

> By the official or planned curriculum is meant what is laid down in syllabuses, prospectuses and so on; the actual or received curriculum is the reality of the pupils' experience. The difference between them may be conscious or unconscious, the cause of any mismatch being either a deliberate attempt by the teachers or others to deceive, to make what

they offer appear more attractive than it really is, or merely the fact that, since teachers and pupils are human, the realities of any course will never really match up to the hopes and intentions of those who have planned it.

(Kelly, 1989)

Kelly believes there is a difference between an actual curriculum and a hidden curriculum although he does not explicitly discuss how they differ. However, one interpretation could be that what is learnt via a hidden curriculum is *attitudes and values not planned by teachers as part of the official curriculum*. In order to try to clarify the difference between official, actual and hidden curricula an example is offered in Table 4.1.

Table 4.1 Official, actual and hidden curricula

Taking and recording blood pressures	
Intention of official curriculum	New students should be supervised by qualified staff until competent
Processes and outcomes of actual curriculum	Most of the time new students are unsupervised and do not develop competence
Learning of hidden curriculum	Some new students come to believe that taking and recording accurate blood pressures is not an important part of a nurse's role

In this section an attempt has been made to explore and clarify some interpretations of what a hidden curriculum is, while accepting Meighan's (1986) assertion that the concept is very ambiguous. The following section will add a little flesh to the foregoing discussion by examining some of the messages and strategies of a hidden curriculum.

Hidden curriculum: messages and strategies

'Teaching is a political activity. Embedded in teaching are the hidden messages about what is valued, what learning is about, and who is in power, in control, and on top' (Bevis and Murray, 1990). In this section the strategies used by students to cope with the demands of school/college life will be explored, together with the messages transmitted via hidden curricula. As a general introduction the classic works of Jackson (1968) and Holt (1969) will be considered.

Jackson asserts that school is a place where children learn to live in a crowd and cope with delay, denial, interruption, and social distraction. Delay is experienced, for example, in queues for scarce resources: 'Only one student at a time can borrow the big scissors, or look through the microscope, or drink from the drinking fountain, or use the pencil sharpener. And broken pencil points and parched throats obviously do not develop one at a time or in an orderly fashion' (Jackson, 1968). Children also learn to be evaluated, receiving praise or reproof, and to experience a clear distinction between the weak (themselves) and the powerful (teachers). Most children, according to Jackson, learn to adapt to the teacher's authority and to listen and look when told to. However, certain practices may be used to cope with the unequal power relationships; for example, 'creating a good impression' or hiding words and actions that might displease the authorities (Jackson, 1968). Jackson recognises that there is a conflict between the habits of obedience and docility engendered in the classroom and the qualities of curiosity and a questioning spirit which are required by scholarship. Yet he believes both can be mastered by the same person, and in any case he considers that the learning of obedience and docility help to prepare children for adult working life.

Jackson thus overall seems to view hidden curriculum as an essentially benign concept. In contrast, Holt (1969) believes that schools foster bad strategies and create fear so that most children fail to develop their creative potential. He describes various strategies used by children to cope with the system: 'mumble, guess-and-look, take a wild guess and see what happens, get the teacher to answer his own questions'. These, Holt believes, are games all humans (adults and children) play when others sit in judgement on them. Fear, according to Holt, is another feature of school life and he suggests that most of the intellectual and creative capacity of children is destroyed by making them afraid: 'afraid of not doing what other people want, of not pleasing, of making mistakes, of failing, of being *wrong*. Thus we make them afraid to gamble, afraid to experiment, afraid to try the difficult and the unknown' (Holt, 1969).

It is interesting to note that some aspects of schooling described by Jackson (1968) and Holt (1969) appear similar to those occurring in higher education. For convenience the following discussion relating to older students, including nurses, will be presented in five interrelated areas: curriculum content and organisation; staff-student interactions; assessment; educational resources; organisational structures.

Curriculum content and organisation

Timetables

Eisner (1985) suggests that school programmes reflect to students the significance of different subject areas and that students learn to read the 'value code'. Cornbleth (1990) asserts that programmes provide opportunities for learning some subjects but reduce opportunities for learning others, and thus communicate what is to be taken seriously by teachers and students. The timing and sequencing of subjects also indicate their relative worthwhileness. Thus one could hypothesise that if student nurses only had, say, four hours in three years devoted to the ethics of health care, and these were timetabled on a Friday afternoon, this could suggest that ethics was of only marginal importance to nurses. Partridge (1983) describes a nursing curriculum which required fewer than 30 hours on such subjects as the health-illness continuum and communications; 100 hours for practice of nursing; 160 hours for medicine and related nursing practice; and 130 hours for surgery and related nursing practice. All this indicates that general nurses need to know very little about health but a great deal about medical and surgical illness (Partridge, 1983).

This is reinforced by the students' clinical experience: medical, surgical, paediatric, operating theatre and recovery room nursing are compulsory; psychiatric and community nursing are optional; rehabilitation and geriatric nursing are not mentioned.

Partridge also highlights the interesting issue of who teaches which subjects. The regulations governing this state that only first aid and the practice of nursing may be taught by someone with no qualifications other than 'basic registration'. 'Thus, the more senior teachers are often allocated subjects such as anatomy and physiology, while more junior staff members teach nursing practice. The message in terms of the knowledge hierarchy is inescapable' (Partridge, 1983).

The theme of timetabling is also discussed by Treacy (1987). In her research study she found that in the Preliminary Training School (PTS) out of all subjects, the most time was allocated to anatomy and physiology. Often this amounted to more than an hour a day, while nursing was left for students to read in their own time. This resulted, Treacy suggests, in the students identifying anatomy and physiology as being 'at the heart of nursing'. Interestingly, Treacy also notes that often, when study periods appeared on the timetable, they were used to fill odd gaps in the day's programme rather than forming part of a study plan.

One could argue that this could transmit subtle messages to students about the value placed on independent study in the curriculum. Further insights on possible messages of the hidden curriculum can be gathered from Clinton's (1982; 1983) participant observation study of two psychiatric nurse training schools. Clinton (1983) suggests that the titles of the sessions in the programme emphasise the routines and rules associated with nursing care, for

Table 4.2 Probing the hidden assumptions of timetables

1. Who is involved in timetabling?
   - (Senior teachers? All teachers? Students?)
2. Who gives timetabled sessions?
   (Students, doctors, teachers, staff from clinical areas?)
   - What is the perceived relative importance of the different contributors?
   - Are there any groups of students who are always taught by the least experienced staff?
3. What is timetabled, how often and when?
   - Are there any 'Cinderella areas' which seem to get the worst slots in the timetable and is this appropriate?
   - Are there any subjects/issues/experiences missing from the timetable?
   - Is the balance of the timetable appropriate and do the titles of the sessions transmit the image of nursing intended by the college?
   - Are any private study sessions included?
4. What view of knowledge is embodied in the timetable?
   (Fragmentation? Integration?)
5. How long are the sessions?
   (Standardised? Any flexibility?)
   - Do students and teachers get a break during longer sessions?
6. Do the answers to 1–5 differ according to the different groups of students, and if so can this be justified?
7. Are all the answers in accordance with the college's philosophy?

example: 'reporting accidents' and 'ordering medications and supplies'. He also states that the 'timetabling arrangements implied that what passed for knowledge in the classroom, topics taken directly from the General Nursing Council's syllabus, had priority over student nurses learning practical skills' (Clinton, 1982).

The foregoing examples may appear rather extreme but they do point to the need for vigilance in the formulation of timetables! As Meighan (1986) asserts, timetables are taken-for-granted facets of school culture, and rarely are their hidden assumptions examined. Meighan poses a number of questions which could help nurse educators probe some of their assumptions. These questions are presented in an expanded and freely adapted form in Table 4.2.

Staff-student interactions

In the previous section of the chapter, students were portrayed as rather passively 'soaking up' messages from timetables. This section involves a shift in focus in which students are portrayed as actively coping with the demands of organisations.

Making a good impression

The strategies students may use are described in several studies including that of Olesen and Whittaker (1968). This study examined the professional socialisation of nurses, and the authors describe the concept of 'studentship' which functions to suggest answers to a perpetually problematic issue: how to get through school with the greatest comfort and the least effort, preserving oneself as a person, while at the same time being a success and attaining the necessities for one's future life' (Olesen and Whittaker, 1968). For these students legitimate power lay with the faculty, and the only path to becoming a professional was defined as 'getting through nursing school'. It was therefore in the students' interests to 'look enthralled in a classroom or appropriately nursely on a ward' (Olesen and Whittaker, 1968). The student also realised that since faculty expected some mistakes it was good policy to admit to some, but such admissions needed to be balanced with many instances of good nursing care of which the instructors had been made aware. Students had to 'blend the correct mixture of assertiveness, humility and awkwardness' (Olesen and Whittaker, 1968).

The importance of making a good impression is also discussed in Becker et al.'s (1961) study of student culture in a medical school. Students, for example, would try to get clues from staff about right answers without revealing their real ignorance by having to say 'I don't know'. Thus one medical student said:

> 'You really learn how to handle these teachers. That's one thing you do learn, so that even if you don't know the answer you can get around them. We certainly learn that very well even if we don't learn anything else.
> (Becker et al., 1961)

Some students believed that their best efforts to make a good impression would not avail and that the safest strategy was to make as little an impression as possible: 'I don't want to make any impressions on anyone. I don't want anybody to know who I am. Dr Lackluster – that's who I want to be. Just as long as I get out of here' (Becker et al., 1961).

The strategy of 'keeping a low profile' was also noted by Treacy (1987) in her qualitative study of General Nurse Training. New students were told that if they did not measure up to standards they would go, and Treacy suggests that all students believed having to leave was

> a possibility to the extent that they felt the need to 'fit-in', 'avoid hassle and notice', generally, 'keep a low profile' and 'study hard and pass examinations'. In the course of these experiences the student learns of her own low status in the hospital hierarchy and of her own powerlessness
>
> (Treacy, 1987)

The importance to students of 'fitting in' is also highlighted in Melia's (1987) study of the occupational socialisation of student nurses. Meeting the expectations of the ward staff meant first and foremost fitting in with the way the ward sister organised her ward. As one student explained: 'even before you begin to think about the patients and how you are going to treat the patients you begin to think – 'just as long as I settle into the ward; get on with the staff' (Melia, 1987).

Discussion with other students is, of course, one way of finding out how best to 'fit in':

> I had heard of the junior probationer's position in the acute diphtheria ward, and of the much-dreaded sister and ward-maid, the latter, in a way, being, as far as the probationers were concerned, as much head of the ward as the former . . . I was given much sympathy and advice by nurses who had had their 'turn', and, principally, was warned not to upset the ward-maid. It was diplomacy, I was told, to avoid 'putting her in her place'.
>
> (*Nursing Mirror*, 1912)

The complex nature of the interactions between ward staff and students is well described by Melia (1987). Students she interviewed seemed to describe a set of unwritten rules which, if followed, enabled them to behave in a way which was acceptable to the ward staff. Thus students were expected to work quickly, 'pull their weight' and to 'look busy' if there was no work to be done. Students often stated that the permanent ward staff did not regard talking with patients as nursing work. The unwritten rules were enforced by subtle means:

> from the looks you get, if things are out of place they just look at you, just find out not from asking anybody, it's just there somehow, you just know it – that's accepted and that's it. People sometimes emit it so strongly that you know that you don't do that sort of thing.
>
> (Melia, 1987)

From an educational viewpoint the findings of these studies are disturbing. For although students are portrayed as *actively* coping with the demands of their situations there is a strong element of social control present, and some aspects of the staff-student relationships militate against the sort of learning which promotes good patient-client care and the personal development of students. In a climate so lacking in openness students are less likely to report errors or admit to lack of understanding and the unwritten rule to work quickly and get through the work can be frankly dangerous. As Ashworth and Morrison (1989) point out, 'some deleterious norms can be appropriated in the same way that valuable and adaptive ways of acting are. A good example is the way corners are cut during dressing procedures to ensure all the early staff's work is completed before the late shift comes on duty' (Ashworth and Morrison, 1989).

One wonders whether some of Gott's (1984) findings of bad practice among students were related to a felt need to 'get through the work quickly' to avoid disapproval from the ward staff. Three students, for example, admitted that when taking blood pressures they 'still couldn't hear it; [they] just wrote down what it was before' (Gott, 1984). It could also be argued that the importance of 'fitting in' could result in some students learning via a hidden curriculum to become passive and compliant practitioners. Thus the often difficult tasks of improving practice and rooting out bad practice could be made more problematic. As one of the clinical teachers in Gott's study stated in relation to the stresses of new students: 'From the very beginning they are not encouraged to express an opinion or ask and question, and no matter how much integrity they've got, there are very few who have the courage to stand out in a crowd'.

Besides receiving tacit messages about the role of a nurse which may conflict with the 'official' image of a professional practitioner, students may also come to acquire a view of *nursing* which was not intended by nurse teachers. Gott (1984), for example, found that the way skills were taught and sequenced was often fragmented and in conflict with the concept of total patient care. Moreover, Gott contends that though students initially seem to recognise that nursing involves relating to people, they quickly learn that for qualified staff, doing things for or to patients is more valued than talking to them. Thus students come to perceive 'real' nursing as doing things to patients.

The above discussion suggests that the interactions between staff and students (and the way the work of the wards is organised) can convey messages to students of a distinctly non-educative nature. Gott makes a number of recommendations which could help reduce these potentially harmful influences. For example, she stresses the importance of nurse teachers showing students alternative acceptable practices rather than focusing on one 'right' school way of doing things. One could argue that ensuring nurses *understand the principles of care* would help them make safe decisions about priorities. Gott also suggests that nurse teachers should draw more upon qualified clinical staff to help in teaching, as well as teaching and practising on the wards themselves.

Teaching methods is another area for improvement identified by Gott (1984). In her study she found that the teaching methods used were more suited to the development of bureaucratic behaviour patterns, and she recommended changes in both teaching methods and teacher-learner relationships. These points will be developed later in this chapter. The need for nurses to develop assertiveness skills is becoming increasingly recognised but students still need support in coping with the pressures of a physically, intellectually and emotionally demanding course of preparation. This support normally comes from teachers and clinicians, but the added external support of a professional student organisation can increase confidence and critical awareness.

The focus of this section has been upon students actively adopting *strategies* to create a good impression and survive in the system. In the next part of the chapter the emphasis shifts to the sort of *messages* students may receive from language.

Hidden messages of language

Walker and Meighan (1986) suggest that language serves different functions: communication, social interaction, control and thought. Unfortunately language can all too easily be used in a way that controls students and discourages thought. Barnes (1969), for instance, suggests that if teachers ask many factual questions they transmit a covert message to students that information is more important than original thought (cited by Stubbs, 1976).

De Tornyay and Thompson (1987) cite a study by Scholdra and Quiring (1973) who analysed the type of questions asked by nursing instructors in clinical conferences at a baccalaureate school of nursing. During 22 conferences the instructors asked 617 questions but only six of these were higher order questions involving analysis, synthesis and evaluation. Eaton et al. (1977) analysed 13,046 observations of micro-teaching sessions involving nurse educators, and identified a number of discussion-stopping behaviours. For example, teachers may allow insufficient time for students to answer questions. Thus after a minimal pause teachers may answer their own questions or rephrase them rather than allowing time for thoughtful responses (Eaton et al., 1977). In the context of a hidden curriculum, it could be argued that such teacher behaviour conveys covert messages to students that thinking is not an important activity. House et al. (1990) suggest how questioning can contribute to more effective teaching, and those teachers who wish to examine this aspect of their practice more closely could find it helpful to tape-record and analyse one or two teaching sessions. Such an analysis could focus not only on the form and content of questions but also on the extent to which all students' contributions are valued. This is an aspect of teaching which will be explored further in the following section.

Labelling and teacher expectations

Meighan (1986) suggests that 'the central proposition in studies of teacher expectations is that pupils tend to perform as well or as badly as their teachers expect'. Thus a teacher might label a pupil as bright or dull, convey in possibly unintended ways his or her expectations of that pupil, and this could influence the pupil's subsequent progress. Meighan includes summaries of some interesting studies relating to teacher expectations. For example, Garwood and McDavid's (1975 study cited by Meighan, 1986 suggested that teachers had stereotypes related to children's first names. Thus boys called David were seen as having positive qualities such as strength and wisdom, while the name Harold was associated with characteristics such as weakness and foolishness. Burns (1982) cites Brophy and Good's (1974) review of the research literature of teacher expectations, and suggests that these studies 'demonstrate irrevocably that teachers treat individual students differently and in ways that are often self-defeating'. It is important to note, though, that the effects of teacher expectations upon pupils' self-concepts are stronger in younger children. Older students are less exposed to one teacher's influence and are better equipped to judge a teacher's credibility. The impact of teacher expectations (high or low) on mature students' performance may therefore be reduced (Burns, 1982).

However, even if one accepts this, it could be argued that teachers who convey negative messages to students, for *whatever* reason, are likely at the very least to make the educational process less pleasant and satisfying for those students. For this reason it is worth considering Burns' analysis of how teachers convey their perceptions of pupils in verbal and non-verbal ways, and how negative effects can be avoided.

Burns suggests that probably without realising it, some teachers react unequally with pupils, giving positive feedback to some, negative to others, and neglecting yet others. He stresses the need for teachers to interact evenly with all pupils, and to talk with all pupils including those quiet students who can easily be ignored. Eble (1988) recognises that teachers probably do not like all of their students equally, but he argues 'that should not prevent us from treating students fairly, making ourselves available to all, being sensitive to inadvertent slighting and favouring, and being receptive and understanding rather than defensive when a student, for whatever reasons, feels discriminated against'.

The importance of non-verbal communication cannot be overemphasised, and as Burns (1982) points out a teacher's indifferent manner, forced smile and tightly crossed arms may convey more clearly than words the message 'I don't care for you'. By contrast, a warm tone of voice, friendly smile and eye contact all convey messages that the student is accepted. Positive messages can also be conveyed by using students' names and by referring back to the contributions of individuals in discussions. With regard to questions by teachers, Eble (1988) suggests that 'Enthusiasm for all responses, not just for right answers, is both a courtesy and an incentive'. The practice of at least occasionally giving out handouts personally to students provides an opportunity for a fleeting interaction with every member of a group. Moreover, with longer sessions involving groupwork, messages of trust may be conveyed to students if, instead of the whole class having a set coffee or tea break together, groups break when necessary for refreshment, working in their own way before reconvening at a prespecified and negotiated time for the plenary session.

In these ways teachers can help to convey positive regard and expectations to all students, whatever their abilities and regardless of whether such students are equally likeable. Yet having said this, it is all too easy to label students or groups of students as 'bright', 'lively', 'difficult', 'moaners' and so on. Indeed, as Hargreaves (1975) points out, there is a universal human need to place people in categories. The danger of categorising students, however, is that categories can become fixed and for this reason Hargreaves suggests that teachers should try to avoid making categorisations which are 'premature or too sharp and final'. They should also be constantly open to the possibility of re-categorising students, and should be careful about staff-room gossip and student records, both of which can be used to support a categorisation and make it static. For even if adult students are less likely to accept a label, and a self-fulfilling prophecy is less probable, nevertheless one could speculate that when teachers make static negative categorisations of students, learning experiences are less likely to be fruitful and enjoyable. This possibility is explored further in the next part of the chapter which focuses on the educational experiences of students who are black or from minority ethnic groups.

Cottle (1978) cites the school experiences of a West Indian boy called Lanny:

I went to school three years with a bunch of kids, none of 'em could read. Black kids, white kids, none of 'em could read. So they put us in this class together, man, where there was supposed to be special help for us, just in reading, you understand. We got, I don't know, maybe twenty five kids in that room. Room used to smell too, man, 'cause it was right next to the kitchen. They used to keep all the extra tables and chairs in there, but then they cleared it out for us, all of us being the special cases. You want to know what happens? First thing they get is a white teacher, and she ain't old, man, she's Queen Victoria's grandmother! And we're the first blacks she has ever seen in her life. But you think she says something about it? Oh no, she's real cool about it. She gives us seats where we have to sit and doesn't it come out whites over there and us over here? Okay, I can take that. I say to myself, well, she ain't going to be no close friend, man, but maybe the old lady's going to help me read. That's a joke, man. A *joke*! She has us reading books out loud, right? She makes the white kids read and they go on and on and on. Then comes us, and what does she do? She listens to us two seconds and says, 'That's wonderful, Lanny,' and goes on to the next one. Two seconds later, 'That's wonderful, Snaker.' Two seconds later, 'That's wonderful, Elaine.' She never hears us for more than a minute, man. So who do you guess got anything out of that special class, man? Wasn't us, I can tell you for sure.

But now I'll tell you something about her, and this is all happening when I was nine, but I knew it then, man, we all knew it then. That woman never knew she was doing it, man. You would have asked her, maybe she'd tell you she treats us all the same but for some reason the white kids just do better than the black kids. Can't tell you why that is, but they do. Maybe it's their home life, you know. That woman never once saw what she was doing, and I'm not sure the white kids did either. But the black kids did. Fact is, *that's* what I learned in that special class. First, I learned that blacks didn't stand a chance with her so we'd none of us get to read properly, and the second thing was that you can't learn nothing in a room next to the kitchen. It smells too much, makes it so you can't think.

(Cottle, 1978)

One of the significant features of this account is that the discrimination appeared to be hidden from the teacher, and possibly from the white children too. However, this study is now over fifteen years old and it related to children not adult students. Of more significance to this discussion of hidden curricula in nursing education are the current educational experiences of black student nurses and those from minority ethnic groups. In order to gain some insights into students' perspectives the writer interviewed small groups of Project 2000 students from several different locations. The analysis which follows is based on a discussion with eight students from one college.

There was a feeling, expressed by some of the group, that black students and those from some minority ethnic groups were regarded by some white people as being less intelligent than English students:

some fail to realise that we are just as intelligent – it's not, you know, we say we are *better* than . . . In some cases people fail to recognise we are just as intelligent in our seminar groups.

Several examples were cited by the students which indicated that in some cases their contributions in seminars were not valued by white people. (It was unclear whether this included teachers or peers, or both.)

you don't feel inclined to participate seeing as, if you have a vital contribution, it's just being neglected and someone else was to make the same point and then they were to take it on board. Then you really wouldn't feel, as I said, inclined to comment or participate as much.

They comment after your contribution, 'Oh, yes, is that so? Yes, oh' [said in an offhand way]. They treated [the Chinese students] really bad. They think they're all stupid . . . When they're in the seminar group if one of the Orientals has anything to say, they're just, er, like [dismissive gesture] shut up, you know . . . so some of them don't say anything at all in the seminar group . . . they tend to stay mum . . . They have one of them, she talks a lot, right, because she is intelligent, she has a degree and stuff like that, and they treat her like a fool, [pause] you know. So the others . . . just stay quiet.

Two Irish students had experienced the odd 'thick Paddy' sort of remark from peers.

You get that quite often 'thick Paddy' . . . and . . . 'that's a very Irish thing to do', it really bugs me. 'That's very Irish' you know, if you say something that's maybe a bit silly, could be a bit silly or somebody else says, . . . an English person, whatever, they just say . . . that's very Irish' . . . that's something that really annoys me.

One black student described in detail an incident in a discussion which indicates the need for teachers to be ever vigilant in ensuring all students are treated equally:

> I raised a point and I wanted to, like, back up the point. He [the teacher] had given us a pamphlet and it so happened he had his . . . I asked him if, you know, could I borrow your pamphlet, please, to, you know, quote the point and so on. And he said, 'I don't have it.' I mean it was there, he said, 'No, I don't have it.' And so I went on and made my point, and it so happened that another girl who was in my group, she happened to be white, a white girl, she wanted to make a point and she just say, you know 'Could I borrow it?' And he took it and held it to her like this [demonstrated] you know he just said 'Look' . . . I mean I was really embarrassed, asking him and he saying no, he doesn't have it and there it was she asking him and he just fetched it out and give it to her, you know . . . and I don't know if he saw my face really drop . . . And then he said, 'Well . . . if you want to, oh, if you want to see it, go and sit with [other student] so you can see it.' And because I always contribute to the whatever, seminar, so I did went across and look it up and substantiated the point I was making but in this case it was very blatant, it was. I mean, and not as if I alone, you know was thinking this way, all the others . . . Why did he treat me so? If he didn't give it to me why say he doesn't have it and when someone else asks, give it to them? He must think about the implications, even if he has forgot or something like that, he could think about what's he's doing.

Another student gave a poignant account of a ward placement experience:

> *Student*:   I was, I was in the ward . . . and I can, I could feel the staff got different attitudes to the other British, um, friend, my friend, she was with me, and they treat me differently and um, it was hard, I couldn't understand why, but maybe, um, they were more friendly to her, maybe because they they was thinking, they've got more things in common, something like that.
> *Author*:   How did the extra friendliness show itself?
> *Student*:   They were talking to her more. If we were sitting together they were coming to her and talking, start talking, talking to her, rather than to me, and um [pause] yes, just . . .
> *Author*:   How did that make you feel?
> *Student*:   Absolutely terrible. I mean I was feeling, um, first, just left out, why they don't talk to me, or what's wrong with me?

One student was shouted at publicly by a teacher for being late for an appointment and some of the students recalled a 'miserable experience' with a bus driver who swore at two black female students. Another student had already experienced racism from a patient:

> *Student 1*:   A patient called me names already.
> *Student 2*:   That's the worst thing that could happen, that.'

Student 1 then related how she was asked by a nurse to help care for a patient who said, 'I don't want any black people touching me this morning.' The nurse said, 'Ah, she isn't black, you know, she's brown,' to which the student replied, 'Listen, I am black, all right?'

In another incident a member of staff was discussing care of pressure sores:

> We did, um, care of pressure sores and he was saying about, like, a red spot would occur, I mean that is on caucasian skin or white skin and one of the girls had to say, 'What if this is black skin? What would be the symptom or the sign? It must be different.' But he said they never really look into it, so . . . you know the symptoms, in terms of colouring and things like that they would be different, but he said they never really look into that.

Interestingly, Campbell (1990, cited by Carlisle, 1990) reports similar experiences in her training, and she suggests that when nurses are not taught about caring for people from different minority ethnic groups it 'tells students that the people who set the curricula see Britain as a nation with only one colour of skin'. It also marginalises black students.

The writer's discussion with the group of Project 2000 students, however, suggests that worthwhile curricular changes can be sabotaged by some white peers:

> And when we have lectures about racism and . . . different cultures, British people are not interested at all . . . they're not interested . . . because they were talking and laughing and they weren't paying attention and they were disturbing those who wanted to listen.

Another comment highlighted the importance of colleges having an equal opportunities policy which ensures the formulation of their criteria as to how branch placements are made. One student was concerned because she had come to realise that there were more 'black and ethnic minority groups' in the 'mental handicap or psychiatric unit', and she had wondered why this was so. The writer asked if anyone else in the group would like to comment on this, and one student said:

> we had to put which branch we want to do . . ., like me I put Adult or Children. So if they see that there are so many people in Adult, what she is saying is the whites will be put in Adults, or Children, the blacks will be pushed into Mental Health or Mental Handicap. So that's . . . the line of demarcation there. It's not, like, attributing merit, it's just the colour of their skin that's being considered.

Finally, the students suggested ways in which the situation for black students and those from minority ethnic groups could be improved. The suggestion was made that people need to know their geography and make sure they know students' ethnic origins. This would stop infuriating mistakes in which, for example, students from India and Pakistan are regarded as having the same ethnic origins. Another student stressed the need for a broad knowledge of different cultures, rather than focusing on the English cultures, since 'nurses come in contact with different people'. Furthermore,

> Nurse tutors and so on, they have to be genuinely interested in us as student nurses and don't just see colours and don't have expectations or stereotype. It shouldn't be so. Get to know everybody as a person . . . so . . . can help them.

In a similar vein a student remarked:

> I know the tutors are talking about holistic care, and they're trying to explain to us what holistic care means. I think we must tell some of them . . .

The strength of feeling was expressed thus by one student:

> And what we are saying is that, actually we have respect for other people that is not mutual. It's very embarrassing sometimes. So, sometimes you have to . . . hold it inside yourself because one day, I mean, it can burst out, so it can end very tragically.

The preceding discussion involved only eight students and in no way could one generalise from their comments. Yet the growing body of literature leaves no doubt that racism exists in nursing (King Edward's Hospital Fund for London, 1990), and there is certainly a need for research into how negative messages are transmitted to students, and how the situation can be improved. Change, as Golding (1990) points out, is best seen as an evolutionary process both within the nursing profession and broader social groups. However, she suggests a number of ways in which individuals can contribute to the process of change. These include avoiding negative racial stereotypes and jokes based on prejudice, and listening to the concerns of nurses from black and minority ethnic groups. For clinical and tutorial staff it would seem crucial to provide a forum for students to discuss openly any racist incidents they experience in their work, and to receive support. One way of developing curricula in nursing education would be to adopt the concept of transcultural nursing (Leininger, 1978, cited by Weller, 1991). Transcultural nursing relates cultural and anthropological knowledge to nursing theory and practice in order to help the nurse understand behaviours which may seem illogical from the nurse's own cultural viewpoint (Weller, 1991). Finally, in order to try to uncover any hidden messages which tend to devalue students and their culture, teachers could include specific items on module/course evaluation forms, for example:

1. To what extent have you felt valued as a person on the course?
2. To what extent has your culture been valued on the course?

In this section a range of hidden messages relating to staff-student interactions have been discussed. Such interactions are also important in the area of assessment.

The assessment of students

Ramsden (1988) suggests that probably 'the most significant single influence on students' learning is their perception of assessment'. For this reason it is important to explore those aspects of assessment which may form part of a hidden curriculum. Becker et al. (1968) studied undergraduate life at the University of Kansas from the students' perspectives and one of the areas examined was academic work. Finding out what teachers wanted in assessments and giving it to them was a crucial survival strategy, for:

> They [instructors] don't like for you to have a different interpretation than the one they think is right . . . It doesn't pay to disagree with them
> (Becker et al., 1968)

Becker et al. concluded that:

> given the importance of grades and the total control by faculty over the terms of their distribution, students cannot act as autonomous intellectuals, cannot pursue learning for its own sake, but must seek information on faculty behavior, present and prospective, before they can plan what they will do. In this sense, the relationship of subjection works against the commonly stated faculty goal of training students to be intellectually free and self-directing
> (Becker et al., 1968)

A similar conclusion is reached by Snyder (1973) who explores the dissonance between the messages coming from formal curricular intentions, and the other contradictory messages associated with the strategies students find they must use to obtain academic rewards. Finding out what to learn and how to learn it so as to achieve high grades, forms part of a hidden curriculum which can stifle creativity and make the relationship between student and teacher competitive rather than co-operative (Snyder, 1973). Davis' (1975) study of the professional socialisation of student nurses demonstrated the importance they attached to 'psyching out' their instructors, but Davis noted too that:

> in trying to divine in a calculating fashion the wishes of a superior seemingly for the sole purpose of gaining academic rewards which it is in her power to bestow, students occasionally catch glimpses of themselves as amoral manipulators, as persons prepared to discredit convictions which have formed part of their innermost selves
> (Davis, 1975)

Miller and Parlett's (1974) study of university students is important because it highlights individual differences in students' approaches to assessment. First, there were 'cue conscious' students who talked about the need to be perceptive to 'cues' from staff about, for example, examination topics, aspects of the subject favoured by the staff and whether they were making a good impression in a tutorial. A smaller group of students were not only perceptive to cues but *actively* tried to interact with staff and create a good impression with them. They made deliberate attempts to find out about examinations questions and the interests of their oral examiner. Miller and Parlett (1974) called this group of students 'cue-seekers'. The third and largest group were neither perceptive nor active and were labelled by Miller and Parlett as 'cue-deaf'. Whereas the cue-conscious and the cue-seekers regarded their strategies as very important for success, the cue-deaf regarded working as hard as they could as the ingredient for success. Miller and Parlett compared the students' final degree class with their cue type and found that the cue-conscious and cue-seekers tended to get better degree classes than the cue-deaf.

One cannot help but be dismayed by the impoverished student-teacher relationships apparent in some of the literature relating to hidden curricula of assessment, and with the way systems can operate to make students' experiences far from educational. Indeed, as Ramsden (1988) points out, it is the context of learning – the student's subjective perception of the requirements of teachers – that is the force driving much of their learning. Unfortunately, however, students' perceptions of what teachers reward may lead those students to adopt learning approaches which do not enable qualitative changes in understanding to occur (Ramsden, 1988). A surface approach to learning, for example, is associated with the memorisation of information, procedures for assessment, and knowledge is cut off from everyday reality. The student's intention is to complete task requirements. A deep approach to learning involves, for instance, relating concepts to everyday experience, distinguishing between evidence and argument and organising and structuring content. The student's intention is to understand (Ramsden, 1988).

Boud (1990) summarises some research findings on the relationship between assessment and learning in higher education and it paints a bleak picture. For example, it appears that successful performance in examinations may not indicate that students have a good grasp of concepts which were supposed to be tested. Boud concludes that in spite of the good intentions of staff, 'assessment tasks are set which encourage a narrow, instrumental approach to learning that emphasises the reproduction of what is presented, at the expense of critical thinking, deep understanding and independent activity'. Boud stresses the importance of helping students to develop essential elements of professional practice such as learning how to learn, how to monitor their own work and judge its worth. He suggests various ways in which assessment schemes could be improved. For example, he advocates active monitoring of assessment practices to identify to what extent such practices encourage meaningful learning and an understanding of key concepts. Interestingly, Altschul and Sinclair's (1989) qualitative analysis of examination systems in pre-registration education in Scotland showed that there were high failure rates on questions dealing with concepts central to nursing such as communication, pain, teamwork or bereavement. Where possible students avoided such questions (Altschul and Sinclair, 1989). Boud

(1990) also advocates monitoring students' perceptions of actual assessment since it is these perceptions which govern students' behaviour. In addition, he recommends reviewing assessment schemes to see if they adequately reflect the decision-making processes required by practitioners (Boud, 1990). All of these suggestions have implications for course/module evaluation in nursing education.

Boud draws on the work of Donald Schön in relation to reflective practice, and claims that assessment practices can lock us into a narrow conception of preparation for practice. Schön (1983, 1987 cited by Boud, 1990) argues that reflection-in-action is a vital element in competent practice; that is, the ability of practitioners to monitor their practice as they do it, and to assess what they need to do, drawing upon both their tacit knowledge and technical skills. Boud (1990) suggests that journals could be used as a way of assessing reflective practice. Journals can facilitate self-assessment, and this, together with peer-assessment can help students to take responsibility for their own learning and to form sound judgements about their work.

Boud's recommendations could help to reduce some of the adverse effects of a hidden curriculum in relation to assessment. Contract grading is another approach which could reduce the dominance of grades and what Eble (1988) calls the 'Whadyget syndrome'! An example of an A-grade contract at the McMaster University School of Nursing can be found in the work of Knowles (1986). Small investigative studies and suitably challenging essay titles and can give students opportunities to exercise their creativity and critical thinking skills, but probably most students need help in becoming less dependent on teachers. Moreover, in trying to adopt new approaches to assessment, teachers may be constrained by a shortage of resources, such as library facilities.

Educational resources: more hidden messages

Library and information services

Shepherd and Yeoh (1990) point out that College of Nursing Libraries are traditionally weak in subjects such as philosophy, ethics, sociology, psychology, politics and environmental issues, yet these are the areas Project 2000 students need to study. However, a survey of Project 2000 colleges indicated that in five of the 13 colleges no additional library funding was available. Moreover, multi-site colleges, created by the amalgamation of a number of smaller colleges, posed particular problems, for example in distribution of resources and in access of students to those resources. In terms of a hidden curriculum, shortage of books and difficulty in gaining access to them *could* send messages to students that wide reading is not a valued part of education. The study by Shepherd and Yeoh highlights the need for thorough evaluation of library facilities both by the English National Board education officers and also College staff. As Shepherd and Yeoh argue, 'Validating bodies such as the English National Board (ENB) have the opportunity to make a major contribution to raising standards of nursing (library) provision.' It is clearly essential, too, that nurse teachers work closely with librarians both informally, and by ensuring their expertise is utilised in curriculum development groups.

In the next section, this discussion about hidden messages and educational resources will focus on buildings and the environment.

Buildings and the environment

At a Royal College of Nursing student conference, an RGN student complained that when the Project 2000 students started there were videos, computers and new carpets. 'They got bouquets of flowers, and sweatshirts. We didn't even get a cup of coffee. They are making them so special and different' (cited by Tattam, 1991).

This incident shows how in unintended ways messages about relative value can be transmitted to students. Buildings, too, can convey powerful messages. Leaking ceilings and peeling paint, whether these occur in nurses' homes or classrooms, 'tell' students something about how they, and probably their specialty are valued. One thing nurse teachers could do is review the usage of rooms to see whether certain groups of students always have the least pleasant classroom accommodation.

Meighan (1986) notes how the layout of classrooms conveys messages to students about the expected channel of communication. Desks in rows facing the front, for example, suggest a teacher-centred approach. Meighan also includes an interesting section on different layouts of head teachers' offices and the clues about their leadership styles which may emanate from those layouts! In the following section some hidden messages of organisational structures will be discussed.

Organisational structures

In her study Treacy (1987) noted that for tutors and students, the school of nursing replicated the hierarchical structures of clinical areas, and she analyses the structural features of the organisation using Bernstein's concepts of classification and framing. Classification was strong, hence boundaries between theory and practice were strong. Framing was also strong for teachers and students. Hence students had little or no control 'over the selection, organisation and pacing of knowledge transmitted and received in the pedagogical relationship' (Bernstein, 1971, cited by Treacy, 1987). Strong framing may result in students feeling devalued and ignorant and they may become passive, uncritically accepting transmitted information (Treacy, 1987). Teachers, too, were constrained by the 'organization of the school, service demands and a syllabus and examination structure geared to demonstrating knowledge acquired rather than ways of knowing'.

Treacy's research is important, not least because it indicates how messages of subordination, domination and powerlessness can be transmitted to students. The current reform of nursing education will hopefully do much to improve the sort of situation portrayed by Treacy but Project 2000

BELMONT UNIVERSITY LIBRARY

students will still have to function within bureaucratic settings. Moreover, as Treacy emphasises, change in nursing education involves change in a number of different spheres; for example, in the attitudes of all nurses towards their nursing role, their patients and their colleagues. The successful implementation of a continuing education programme for all nurses, midwives and health visitors is clearly of crucial importance if the hopes of Project 2000 are to be fulfilled.

The preceding sections have explored hidden curricula relating to four inter-related areas: curriculum content and organisation; staff-student interactions; assessment; educational resources; and organisational structures. Suggestions have been made as to how the insights drawn from the literature can indicate ways of improving students' educational experiences. In the next part of this chapter, some theoretical approaches to the 'hidden curriculum' and their relevance to nurse teachers will be examined briefly.

Theoretical perspectives on 'the hidden curriculum'

Giroux (1983) discusses three different approaches evident in the literature related to the hidden curriculum. The first approach, characterised by the work of writers such as Jackson (1968), regards the hidden curriculum as a necessary part of socialisation for adult life. This traditional perspective, Giroux (1983) argues, reduces learning to the 'transmission of predefined knowledge' and fails to challenge dominant societal norms and values relating, for example, to racial inequalities. The liberal perspective sees students as more active in the process of schooling, and there is an emphasis on analysing how teachers and pupils create and negotiate classroom meanings. This approach usually ignores, however, the sort of constraints which impinge upon the work of teachers, for example, hierarchical relationships, prevailing ideologies and poor resources. By contrast, the radical perspective on the hidden curriculum focuses on societal influences and constraints upon classroom processes, but in so doing often provides little hope for teachers wanting to counteract inequalities relating to race, gender and so on.

Giroux's three approaches represent ideal types but it would appear that most studies of professional socialisation in nursing, including those mentioned in this chapter, relate to the liberal perspective. Treacy (1987), however, emphasises the importance of examining structural aspects of the educational process in studies of professional socialisation, and in her own research she considered student nurses' subjective experiences in terms of objective reality, i.e. the context of those experiences.

The three theoretical perspectives described by Giroux (1983) provide a useful framework for analysing the literature related to the hidden curriculum, but the intention now is to discuss the relevance of the perspectives for nurse educators and clinicians.

The traditional perspective encompasses a generally benign view of the hidden curriculum, and serves as a useful reminder that norms and values may be *tacitly* transmitted to students in colleges and practice settings. The liberal perspective, with its focus on teacher-student interactions, provides many insights into how teachers and clinical staff can improve educational practice, and this chapter has included some suggestions as to how this could be achieved. The radical perspective stresses the political, social and economic constraints upon teachers in colleges of nursing and midwifery, and clinical colleagues, and provides a blueprint for professional passivity with regard to developments which threaten sound educational practice and patient/client care. A less deterministic and gloomy approach would be to stress the importance of collective action and professional involvement in tackling issues such as equal opportunities at all levels of decision-making.

Implicit in all of the preceding discussion is a belief that teachers and clinical staff should be aware of hidden curricula and should accept some responsibility for what is learnt via hidden curricula. The first problem, however, is to find hidden curricula!

Finding hidden curricula

Cornbleth (1990) argues that we need

> to question or make problematic those aspects of schooling commonly accepted as normal or natural so as to reveal layers of meaning which are not part of our everyday awareness. In other words, our inquiries ought to probe beneath the veneer of supposedly self-evident and self-justifying assumptions and practices . . . Such inquiry is necessarily interpretive as well as material, incorporating participant conceptions and acknowledging our own values.
>
> (Cornbleth, 1990)

Vallance (1980) suggests that in exploring the hidden curriculum we seek an understanding of the *kinds* of learnings occurring via the hidden curriculum, *how* these are communicated to students, *by whom* and possibly *when*. In addition we need to know the educational significance of these covert learnings, and make a decision about what action, if any, we want to take. Probing hidden curricula, according to Vallance, requires the use of qualitative methods of enquiry, and for nurse educators this emphasises the importance of gathering qualitative evaluation data from students. This sort of scrutiny, however, does not go far enough and Cornbleth (1990) would agree with Giroux's (1983) contention that the 'notion of the hidden curriculum (should) also be linked to a notion of liberation, grounded in the values of personal dignity and social justice'.

Taking action

Martin (1976) discusses the question of what we do with a hidden curriculum when we find it. She argues that it is only when a hidden curriculum is harmful – when undesirable beliefs, attitudes, values and behaviours are learnt – that the question of what to do becomes urgent. Rooting out such undesirable learnings though, may be easier said than done, for as Martin points out, such attitudes are likely to be the products of entrenched practices and structures. One line of action for teachers is to raise students' consciousness of hidden curricula so that they are in a better position to resist what is going on. In other words, a critical examination of undesirable learnings received via the hidden curriculum becomes part of the formal nursing curriculum. In order to enable such consciousness-raising and critical scrutiny to take place it is clearly necessary for student teachers and clinical staff to understand the problems and possibilities of hidden curricula. Another strategy open to teachers is actively to encourage the development of positive qualities such as critical thinking, creativity and reflection. This chapter has included suggestions as to how teachers can facilitate truly educational experiences with students. In the last section a worked example is provided to illustrate how a process approach could be used to promote the development of some of those qualities which lie at the heart of good nursing practice.

Developing caring: a process approach

Stenhouse (1975) suggests that a curriculum can be planned by selecting content to exemplify key concepts such as 'causation' in history or 'tragedy' in literature. These concepts are the 'focus of speculation, not the object of mastery'. A key concept in nursing is 'caring', but identifying what exactly caring *is* and how it can be demonstrated is by no means straightforward. One way of respecting students' cultures and their individual differences in the exploration of 'caring', is to ask them to select passages from literature which exemplify *for them* what constitutes caring (or lack of it). The following extract from William Horwood's *Duncton Wood* provides an example of the sort of material which could be used as a basis for discussion:

> Long before (Rose) fully entered the tunnel, she knew that (Bracken) was there. She could smell the heaviness of disease and hear the terrible rasping sound of the very ill. 'Oh, my dearest', she whispered as she entered the tunnel and made her way along it to where she could see Bracken lying. He was huddled to one side of the tunnel, his back paws limp, and his snout and forepaws lost in the darkness ahead. His coat was grimy with dirt and round the terrible wound in his left shoulder were the congealings of blood and the spreading of poison. The tunnel floor about him was grimy with droppings and half-eaten food.
>
> She touched him very, very gently on his good shoulder and whispered softly to him, but he did not respond at all, his breathing short and painful, his eyes closed, his snout bearing the pallor of near-death.
>
> She could see how close to death he was, and how deeply he had suffered. Yet she was puzzled by the fact that the injury itself, though deep and unpleasant, was no worse than many she had seen and from which other moles, surely no fitter than Bracken had been, had recovered without any help at all. Such thoughts were natural to Rose, who treated any mole in trouble by trying to see what were the causes of his distress, knowing that more often than not they were different from what the victims themselves thought they were.
>
> How often had a mole come to her with aches and pains in his shoulders which she had treated by massaging his haunches with comfrey; how often

had she treated a loss of smell, the most terrible affliction for any mole, by buffeting the mole's back? Rose's treatments often seemed bizarre, but they worked.

She suspected that Bracken's illness lay not so much in the wound as in Bracken himself, and perhaps in the way the wound had been inflicted. Clearly, it had been done when he was in a state of distress and weakness . . . well, she couldn't very well ask him.

She began by gently caressing him and grooming his fur, so that slowly she could feel each part of his body relax under her paws and snout until his breathing grew a bit more peaceful and his paws a little less limp. This took her many hours, for he was so weak that she had to be very slow and gentle.

After this she cleaned the wound itself, using juice from the ramson, whose stinging smell also served to purify the air of the tunnel. He groaned a little when she did this, but not much, though he restlessly moved his head from one side to another in his unconsciousness. . .

How long Rose gave herself to the healing of Bracken she never knew, for she was lost to the world as she did it . . .

For three days, perhaps four, (she) stayed tending (him) and cherishing the life in him back to hope and light.

However, the day came when Rose knew that Bracken, though not fully healed, was at least safe . . . His breathing became deeper and more rhythmic, his weak paws now moved restlessly with life, his groans no longer held the agony she had first heard in them. He stirred . . . into consciousness . . . though he did not seem to know that Rose was there with him.

At last she left him, still only on the verge of conscious health again, finding first for him in the tunnels some food which she placed ready at his side. So many times she had left a mole like this, healed as best she knew how but seeming so vulnerable before the rest of the journey into health and wholeness which, finally, they must make for themselves.

(Horwood, 1986)

Darbyshire (1991) argues that 'Establishing caring as a founding concept for nurse education . . . recognises that caring, in its trans-formative, nurturing, empowering and creative sense, must form an explicit foundation for education.' Much of the literature on the hidden curriculum stresses its negative influences and outcomes: impoverished student-staff relationships, fear of failure, task orientation, passivity, and injustice. Perhaps if caring becomes a central curriculum concept and a quality characterising relationships between health professionals, then nurses may be better able to help in the alleviation of suffering and the promotion of wellness, well-being and wholeness.

Acknowledgement

My thanks are due to Brian Dolan of the Royal College of Nursing Association of Nursing Students for his help in the preparation of part of this chapter, to the Project 2000 students who agreed to be interviewed, and to their course tutor and Principal who gave me permission to do so.

References

Alexander, M.F. (1982). Integrating theory and practice: an experiment evaluated. In *Advances in Nursing 4: Nursing Education*. M.S. Henderson (ed.). Churchill Livingstone, Edinburgh, pp. 56–80.

Altschul, A.T. and Sinclair, H.C. (1989). A qualitative analysis of examination questions set for students of nursing in Scotland. *Nurse Education Today*, **9(3)**, 161–71.

Ashworth, P. and Morrison, P. (1989). Some ambiguities of the student's role in undergraduate nurse training. *Journal of Advanced Nursing*, **14(12)**, 1009–15.

Becker, H.S., Geer, B., Hughes, E.C. and Strauss, A.L. (1961). *Boys in White*. University of Chicago Press, Chicago.

Becker, H.S., Geer B. and Hughes E.C. (1968). *Making the Grade*. Wiley, New York.

Bevis, E.O. and Murray, J.P. (1990). The essence of the curriculum revolution: emancipatory teaching. *Journal of Nursing Education*, **29(7)**, 326–31.

Boud, D. (1990). Assessment and the promotion of academic values. *Studies in Higher Education*, **15(1)**, 101–11.

Burns, R. (1982). *Self-concept Development and Education*. Holt, Rinehart & Winston, London.

Carlisle, D. (1990). Trying to open the doors. *Nursing Times*, **86(18)**, 42–3.

Clinton, M. (1982). Training psychiatric nurses: towards a sociological analysis of the hidden curriculum. Part 1. *Nursing Review*, **1(3)**, 4–6.

Clinton, M. (1983). Training psychiatric nurses: towards a sociological analysis of the hidden curriculum. Part 2. *Nursing Review*, **1(4)**, 13–5.

Cornbleth, C. (1990). *Curriculum in Context*. Falmer, London.

Cottle, T.J. (1978). *Black Testimony. The Voices of Britain's West Indians*. Wildwood House, London.

Darbyshire, P. (1991). The American revolution. *Nursing Times*, **87(6)** 57–8.

Davis, F. (1975). Professional socialization as subjective experience: the process of doctrinal conversion among student nurses. *A Sociology Of Medical Practice*, C. Cox and A. Mead (eds), Collier-Macmillan, London, pp. 116–31.

De Tornyay, R. and Thompson, M.A. (1987). *Strategies for Teaching Nursing*, 3rd edn. Wiley, New York.

Eaton, S., Davis, G.L. and Benner, P.E. (1977). Discussion stoppers in teaching. *Nursing Outlook*, **25(9)**, 578–83.

Eble, K.E. (1988). *The Craft of Teaching*, 2nd edn. Jossey-Bass, San Francisco.

Eggleston, J. (1977). *The Sociology of the School Curriculum*. Routledge & Kegan Paul, London.

Eisner, E.W. (1985). *The Educational Imagination*. Macmillan, New York.

Giroux, H.A. (1983). *Theory and Resistance in Education*. Heinemann, London.

Golding, J. (1990). Racism at work. *Nursing Standard*, **4(27)**, 23.

Gott, M. (1984). *Learning Nursing*. Royal College of Nursing, London.

Hargreaves, D.H. (1975). *Interpersonal Relations and Education*. Student edn. Routledge & Kegan Paul, London.

Hargreaves, D. (1980). Power and the paracurriculum. In *Standards, Schooling and Education*. A Finch and P. Scrimshaw (eds). Hodder and Stoughton, Sevenoaks, pp. 126–37.

Holt, J. (1969). *How Children Fail*. Penguin, Harmondsworth.

Horwood, W. (1986). *Duncton Wood*. Arrow Books, London.

House, B.M., Chassie, M.B. and Spohn, B.B. (1990). Questioning: an essential ingredient in effective teaching. *Journal of Continuing Education in Nursing*, **21(5)**, 196–201.

Jackson, P. (1968). *Life in Classrooms*. Holt, Rinehart & Winston, New York.

Jenkins, D. and Shipman, M.D. (1976). *Curriculum: an Introduction*. Open Books, Shepton Mallett.

Kelly, A.V. (1989). *The Curriculum. Theory and Practice*. 3rd edn. Paul Chapman, London.

King Edward's Hospital Fund for London (1990). *Racial equality: the nursing profession*. Equal Opportunities Task Force Occasional Paper No. 6. King Edward's Hospital Fund, London.

Knowles, M. (1986). *Using Learning Contracts*. Jossey-Bass, San Francisco.

Martin, J.R. (1976). What should we do with a hidden curriculum when we find one? *Curriculum Inquiry*, **6(2)**, 135–51.

Meighan, R. (1986). *A Sociology of Educating*, 2nd edn. Cassell, London.

Melia, K.M. (1981). *Student Nurses' Accounts of their Work and Training: A Qualitative Analysis*. PhD thesis, University of Edinburgh.

Melia, K. (1987). *Learning and Working. The Occupational Socialization of Nurses*. Tavistock, London.

Miller, C.M.L. and Parlett, M. (1974). *Up to the Mark*: *a Study of the Examination Game*. Society for Research into Higher Education.

Nursing Mirror (1912). Incident in a nurse's life. A probationer's morning. *Nursing Mirror and Midwives' Journal*, **15**, 20 April 39

Olesen. V.L. and Whittaker, E.W. (1968). *The Silent Dialogue*: *a Study in the Social Psychology of Professional Socialization*. Jossey-Bass, San Francisco.

Opie, I. and Opie, P. (1959). *The Lore and Language of Schoolchildren*. Clarendon Press, Oxford.

Partridge, B. (1983). The hidden curriculum of nursing education. *The Lamp*, **40(7)**, 30.

Ramsden, P. (1988). Studying learning: improving teaching. In *Improving Learning*: *New Perspectives*, P. Ramsden (ed.), pp. 13–31. Kogan Page, London.

Shepherd, T. and Yeoh, J. (eds) (1990). *Resourcing Project 2000 Nursing Courses – the Role of Library and Information Services*. Nursing Information Sub-Group and the Royal College of Nursing Library, London.

Snyder, B.R. (1973). *The Hidden Curriculum*. MIT Press, Cambridge, Massachusetts.

Stenhouse, L. (1975). *An Introduction to Curriculum Research and Development*. Heinemann, London.

Stubbs, M. (1976). *Language, Schools and Classrooms*. Methuen, London.

Tattam, A. (1991). Students warned against Project 2000 bigotry. *Nursing Times*, **87(11)**, 8.

Treacy, M.M. (1987). *'In the Pipeline': a Qualitative Study of General Nurse Training with Special Reference to the Nurse's Role in Health Education*. PhD thesis, Institute of Education, University of London.

Vallance, E. (1977). Hiding the hidden curriculum: an interpretation of the language of justification in nineteenth-century educational reform. In Curriculum and Evaluation, A.A. Bellack and H.M. Kliebard (eds). McCutchan, Berkeley, pp. 590–607.

Vallance, E. (1980). The hidden curriculum and qualitative inquiry as states of mind. *Journal of Education*, **162(1)**, 138–51.

Walker, S. and Meighan, R. (1986). The hidden curriculum of language. In *A Sociology of Educating*, 2nd edn, R. Meighan, Cassell, London, pp. 142–62.

Weller, B. (1991). Nursing in a multicultural world. *Nursing Standard*, **5(30)**, 31–2.

Willis, P. (1977). *Learning to Labour. How Working Class Kids Get Working Class Jobs*. Gower, Aldershot.

5 Political influences in nursing

> If there is one problem facing health care in this country today which prevents the efficient use of ward nursing resources, it is the undervaluing of nursing and nurses.
>
> (Audit Commission, 1991)

The health of a democracy can largely be measured through the existence of a 'civil society' that is, the degree of civic participation at varying levels of decision making (Havel, 1989).

It is ironic that the more involved the citizen is, on an individual basis (and especially when collectively organised) and the more the citizen acts to influence or challenge decisions, the more potentially threatening that individual is seen to be by those in power. The more active the citizen, the more likely they are to be co-opted, or bought off by those in powerful positions.

Too often the state and democracy are thought to be one and the same. But former Prime Minister Margaret Thatcher once said, 'there is no such thing as society'. How then do nurses and midwives exercise citizenship and become, in Trevor Clay's words, 'comfortable with the techniques of politics and the use of power?' (Clay, 1987).

There has been much debate about the role of the nurse in recent years and nursing's leaders have struggled to define that role, in health care terms, in the community and elsewhere. That debate is bound to continue to develop as people of all ages take a keener interest in health care and demand greater choice. Nurses will not be able to reach political maturity and influence in the future without making the connections between what happens in the community, in their wards, and in Whitehall.

In this chapter we attempt to define the political nurse, examine ideas about politics and party politics (commonly confused), as well as internal professional politics. We will touch briefly on the history of nursing and politics, tied in as it is with union politics, and assess the future political context in which nursing is likely to function. The image and culture of nursing and the degree to which this has hindered political development is also taken into account. The role of the nursing regulatory bodies and how they have, with a few exceptions, failed to promote and protect the profession, will also be addressed.

Although education is the subject of another chapter, changes in nursing education are very much a part of nursing's coming of age politically and we will therefore analyse the specific political implications of Project 2000. Economic power is integrally related to education and as cost considerations clearly dominate the health care debate, nurses as well as patients have price tags on their heads.

The political nurse is nowhere more evident than when addressing the question of pay, which reflects her value to the health service and to a society which rewards its workers in economic terms. The clinical grading exercise of 1988 and the mismanagement of its implementation is a perfect illustration of this. Renumeration with local pay deals cannot therefore be ignored.

The tactics and strategy of industrial action in Britain and abroad are assessed as a political tool, as is the oft quoted unwritten pact nurses have with the public; namely that the profession will never let patients suffer. Is the pact, like the British constitution, so flexible that it allows those who already hold power the ability to manipulate it to the disadvantage of the powerless?

A section of this chapter will also examine the media's perception of nursing in parallel with the deference extended and the numerous platforms offered to the medical profession. In addition, the experience of campaigning against the National Health Service (NHS) reforms, which were perceived by many as being 'too little, too late' will be touched on, and a blueprint offered for planning future action locally or nationally.

The issue of health care, as most nurses are aware, has a public resonance that will continue to be seized upon by political parties and used to their political advantage, without necessarily taking into account the nursing perspective.

The promotion of health manifestos and consensus documents are in themselves no substitute for determined, concerted action by specialist groups, for example, midwives, those working in breast care, stoma care, accident and emergency nursing, and care of the elderly, who by harnessing support from consumer groups achieve results. A section of this chapter will deal with motivation and the circumstances which drive a nurse to stand up and be counted, and what happens behind the scenes when they do. Nurses and midwives can encounter conflicts of interest in so many spheres of their work; some are already emerging, namely sponsorship of stoma care nursing posts; the quality equation and profit in private residential and nursing homes, and the use of people with HIV and AIDS for sometimes dubious research.

Finally, we will conclude by outlining a strategy for the future. We suggest that just as nurses and midwives seek to establish standards of care and measure patient outcomes, the political professional or radical clinician should be able to establish standards of citizenship, and be politically responsible. The profession should also be demanding this of its leaders.

Who is the political nurse?

The political nurse is aware and assertive, She makes it her business to inform herself about factors affecting her practice and to avoid feelings of powerlessness by taking action to ensure that unacceptable situations are brought to the attention of those in authority.

Being aware of the appropriate vehicles for political action and thinking through the consequences goes beyond most people's perception of politics.

Politics is seen in terms of casting votes, yet voting is only one small element of political participation and certainly conventional politics, politicians and the curious institutions they inhabit, the political parties, are only one form of participation; often the most static, least imaginative and inaccessible.

Politics does not have to be daunting; we all behave politically every day with the decisions we make and with the judgements, alliances and relationships we form. (The nurse or midwife who discreetly refuses to pander to the whims of a bumptious consultant is behaving politically, just as a colleague who gathers signatures for a petition against health service cutbacks is.)

One of the oldest cliches in the world is that 'politics is the art of the possible'. It is also about having the ability to articulate your concerns, to exert pressure and in doing so to facilitate change. What is not often recognised is that politicians of all shades are conservatives with a small 'c'. They all have a stake in the system.

Change is acceptable to them so long as they remain in control; to manage change, to alter the balance of power to suggest 'there may be another way to do this' and to be innovative are all in themselves a threat to anyone who wants to maintain the status quo. Cognizance of this is vital if the political nurse is not to be deterred by hostility from superiors, or indeed anyone whose power base is challenged.

There are varieties of political action and levels of political activity; in any circumstance it is always necessary to determine what is the appropriate target and what method should be employed. Most nurses become politicised through disputes of one sort or another, whether it be a battle between colleagues over a ward closure, a campaign against the tax community nurses pay on crown cars, or industrial action over pay and conditions. Some people are 'educated' to become political, an area we will explore later.

Political confidence and authority must be derived not only from a familiarity with health care issues and power differentials, but an understanding of structures within which practitioners operate.

Nurses should be making it their business to know local political leaders from councillor level to MPs, shop stewards and other union and professional representatives at regional and national level. Knowing what kind of personality you are dealing with is also essential.

The informal networking as done by male community and business leaders, 'the old boy network' more familiar to women through friendship or family maintenance, is necessary and vital to political life. These skills are not necessarily learned, but can almost be intuitive. Sometimes they are not even recognised by individuals who 'network' everyday! This is a reflection of the lack of value nurses ascribe to themselves and their roles, as Elizabeth Hart, lecturer in department of nursing at Nottingham university points out (Hart, 1991). Her research among nurses at a large teaching hospital illustrates that practitioners;

> 'had to rely on the informal 'underground' aspects of their role to influence medical decision making and to establish a supportive base from which to carry out their work of caring and healing. Much of this 'networking' was carried on out of managerial sight or hearing'.

This underground work Hart refers to is a way of coping without creating a fuss, putting one's neck on the line, or being marginalised.

In nursing circles (even in professional bodies which are publicly promoting being political) the noisy outspoken individual is vilified. Any sort of debate is seen to strike at the heart of the nursing hierarchy, when in fact it is a healthy component of a pluralistic society (see Chapter 1 for historical antecedents for this behaviour).

Setting realistic goals when faced with series of challenges can appear awesome, but tackling the status quo can be exhilarating and eventually becomes second nature. The truly political nurse is one who is able to utilise existing attributes; assessment, diagnosis (yes, nurses do diagnose, although they hate to admit it) management, flexibility, and facilitation.

Ultimately, politics is about having the confidence to insist that nurses' views and the nursing element of health care debates are worthy of representation. Since representation is at the core of the democratic ideal, the surrogates in the form of professional politicians have so far not managed to do a very good job. There can be no substitute for self-advocacy.

In order to reclaim critical thinking and use it in the normal course of nursing work, it has to be practised by a large bulk of the nursing population. Those who remain silent, hiding behind the authority they command in the hierarchy and keeping information from other staff and patients/clients alike, need to have the lid blown off their secret world. Once this is done, being assertive and asking difficult questions will not be something that is the pastime of mavericks and trouble makers, but an everyday activity.

The power of the past

> While nursing has constructed a labyrinth of internal politics, it has proved consistently inept when it has ventured into the area of governmental politics.
>
> (Clay, 1989)

The history of nursing and politics has been intertwined with the profession's perception of, and value for, itself. Nursing has, in the view of many observers remained aloof from conventional politics because of its religious and military origins; in neither field does democratic dissent and discussion come easily (see Chapter 1).

To act politically in terms of self-representation and letting decision makers know about nursing, and critically, the position of the nurse in relation to patients and clients, is crucial. Are nurses enablers or people who contribute to patients' and clients' sense of helplessness? Most nurses were not trade union members until the late 1970s, and the Royal College of Nursing itself, always struggling with a tea party, twin set and pearls image, which it has only now begun to shake off, did not become a certified trade union until 1977. The college had traditionally been a club for managers and educators who until recently, it may be argued, exercised a disproportionate degree of influence on its activities. The 1980s saw a huge increase in the RCN's membership as the traditional Labour party affiliated unions, NUPE (National Union of Public Employees) and COHSE (Confederation of Health Service Employees) had not been able to attract the majority of apolitical nurses. The former was the domain of porters, orderlies and auxiliaries, and the latter remained the stronghold of the largely male domain of psychiatric and mental handicap nursing.

The erosion of traditional trade unions in the 1980s and 1990s led to a flurry of mergers. The amalgamation of the formerly powerful voice of community nursing and health visiting, the HVA (Health Visitors' Association), and the smaller Community Psychiatric Nursing Association, into the giant MSF (Manufacturing Science and Finance Union), are but two examples, not to mention the colossal UNISON, the new union formed with the merger of COHSE, NUPE and NALGO (National Association of Local Government Officers). It is worthwhile considering whether mergers have diminished the political influence of nursing by diverting energy to internal organisational matters, relating to merger survival, or given small specialist groups a more powerful voice.

Yet the RCN continues to grow. Its unique attraction must be a combination of factors; its Royal Charter, its perceived neutrality, and its no strike policy. Much has been written about the benefits of being a member of the largest nursing organisation in the world, but as yet no survey has shown what actually makes people join. There can be no question that its high profile in the late 1980s when government intransigence seemed to have extinguished all practical opposition contributed to its attraction for nurses.

What is clear is that in contrast with other trade unions, the House of Commons and the media, the RCN leadership, its committees and structures, more accurately reflect a gender balance. However, men are still over represented in positions of authority. But in trade unions, nurses have found a voice and they have begun to break out of the arena which has confined them to being a detached and reactive force, or indeed strike fodder, and have learned to act politically.

The new public sector union UNISON will undoubtedly have negotiating weight, but will professional and consumer issues get lost? Will the RCN ultimately become the nursing division of this union, as a COHSE official once gleefully predicted?

In all nursing organisations, serious debate has begun to take place about the image of the profession, management and individual accountability and the effectiveness of the statutory bodies, unheard of and almost treasonable a decade ago. Criticism and healthy disagreement are encouraged by nursing leaders like Christine Hancock who believe the process of dissent and conflict are in themselves beneficial and can contribute to genuine empowerment (Hancock, 1991). It is only when nurses feel able to do this without fear of being let down by their own colleagues, who should be building a supportive and enabling culture, that they can then effectively challenge the political decisions behind cash limiting care, and the use of health issues as a political football; for example, the disgraceful use of the case of Jennifer Bennett's ear in the 1992 General Election campaign.

It may be hard to stop politicians using cases such as this, but they should be encouraged to remember the words of Neil Kinnock, then Labour party leader who said, 'You can't play politics with people's lives' (Kinnock, 1985).

Moving Images

Nurses, because of the way they have been socialised, contribute to the process of making themselves invisible. This happens through omission or trivialisation of their own critical role in covert psychological activities (see Chapter 2). A new language is therefore needed to be able to effectively communicate the importance of nursing work to lay people.

Practitioners cannot even truly act as patients' advocates until they understand and are confident about the historical process which has led them into the pivotal position of being primary care givers in a highly complex health care system.

In 1988, following Health and Social Security Secretary John Moore's announcement that the Government had accepted the Project 2000 proposals, a number of stern articles appeared in the tabloid press and the *The Spectator* magazine (May, 1988) warning that the educational reforms were a dangerous plot to move nurses away from their role of 'soothing fevered brows', which would, by implication, allow the over-education of women simply doing a manual task. The reforms would give nurses ideas above their station: 'Nursing is predominantly a practical craft and only in its farthest and most specialised reaches does it require anything approaching a highly trained intellect.' Presumably the authors overlook the knowledge and skills required to, care for an elderly person with dementia or a person with a learning disability.

Perhaps such journalists should be invited to spend a day with the practitioners! In a masterful example of guilt by overstatement, the article concludes;

> Let no one be in any doubt, despite its learned name, the Royal College of Nursing is a *trade union*. One can no more expect the college to consider the welfare of patients than one can expect the National Union of Railwaymen to consider the convenience of passengers.

Clearly, the work of Jane Salvage (1985) who has written extensively about the image of nursing, had not reached certain quarters of the establishment at that time. There will be an uphill battle to change images such as 'angel' and 'handmaiden', as prominent journalists, Malcolm Dean of *The Guardian*, Andreas Whittam-Smith of *The Independent* and Nial Dickson of the *BBC* acknowledged at a *Nursing Standard* fringe meeting at RCN Congress 1992.

There are much broader sociological questions than we can address here; for example, the difficulty of associating men with caring and questions about whether caring itself is discredited because it is associated with traditionally female and maternal values, and is a vocation for those prepared to accept poor pay.

If, in the need for companies to recruit more women, childcare is seen as a benefit to women and not to men as parents, it is obvious that feminism has not effected enough societal change to alter those perceptions. But through the process of politicisation, nursing can change its image from that of passive dependency to power and authority.

Nurse prescribing is not just about enshrining the obvious in legislation, it is about acknowledging that a great deal of assessment and care is and can be done without reference to a doctor. So, too, the great interest in complementary therapies. It is now apparent that science and its associated practitioners do not have an answer for everything. A holistic approach and the willingness *not* to view individuals from a pathological perspective, is a nursing model, and one that is increasingly being practised by nurses trained in complementary therapies. It is a model that enhances quality of care and yet is often viewed as being dubious.

Inasmuch as nursing itself has suffered labelling as a women's profession, and therefore less worthy of value, the failure to recognise the contribution of black and ethnic minority nurses is nothing short of a scandal. 'Did you see the lady with the lamp?' war artist William Simpson was asked when he returned home from the Crimea. 'No, Miss Nightingale was always busy inside the hospitals across the bay, but there had been another lady, a Mrs Seacole, working on the battlefields' (Alderman, 1991).

A discussion document from RCN (Royal College of Nursing, 1990a) stated that;

> nurses from black and minority ethnic groups are not helped by the fact that although they are mostly female in a predominantly female profession, the majority of senior posts are not held simply by white people, but by white men. Therefore black people are inadequately represented within the management of nursing, a situation which also applies to their representation on professional and statutory bodies.

Not surprisingly, nurses from black and minority ethnic groups are disproportionately employed in the 'cinderella' services of mental health and elderly care. Reflecting their economic status, a higher proportion work night shifts and significantly more work as enrolled nurses. Registered practitioners from black and ethnic minority groups are also more likely to be reported to the UKCC for misconduct.

The Commission for Racial Equality also found they were discriminated against during the clinical grading exercise (Snell, 1992). So it is little wonder that few recommend nursing as a career for young black people (Lee-Cunin, 1989).

For many years the RCN lagged behind NUPE and COHSE in the production of campaigns and information among the membership on sexual and racial equality matters. A concerted effort has been made since 1990, when a special adviser to the general secretary on equal opportunities was appointed. Nurses are only slowly coming to realise that Britain is a multi-cultural and multi-racial society. Despite the full bi-lingualism of the Welsh office and health service materials and publications in Wales, the RCN Welsh Board has almost no literature available in Welsh.

If nurses wish to see their contribution fully recognised they cannot turn their backs on the need to acknowledge the contribution of their colleagues from the black and ethnic minority communities so that they can work together and progress with the same opportunities. The NHS, as the largest employer of women and of black people in Britain, is an ideal place to begin to rectify the injustice that has been endured for so long.

Education – the war within

Nursing and midwifery education has not been immune from the constant political upheavals that have been a feature of life in the health service. Tutors and students have had to withstand a tremendous battering on all fronts as they seek to secure more funding for pre-and post-basic education, and try to sell the most radical shake-up in nursing education for 100 years to a fearful and ignorant profession.

This has come on top of continuous rounds of college amalgamations and extra demands on tutors to get university degrees. One of the most divisive issues for the students was not, as you might imagine the age old problem of being used as cheap labour in the health service, but the imposition of the poll tax.

Project 2000 has been universally hailed as the way forward by the leaders of nursing in the UK. They campaigned hard for it and to their relief in May 1988, after months of delay the then Secretary of State for Health and Social Security John Moore chose the RCN Congress in Brighton to give the reforms the green light. He got, perhaps a little prematurely, a standing ovation for doing so. As Jane Salvage pointed out

> It had all gone perfectly. Keep them hanging on for the verdict on Project 2000, then reveal it to the UKCC just before the RCN Congress, saving the public performance for the opening day at Brighton. This ensured maximum media coverage, kept the TUC health unions at arm's length and enabled a quick get away before the euphoria could turn into cynicism. The RCN may have been right to avoid biting the hand that feeds it, but rolling on its back and waggling its paws in the air was perhaps a little extreme.
>
> (Salvage, 1988)

The package would 'come with strings', she predicted. Mr Moore's announcement made no mention of money, and by the time the bidding system was set up for the first sites, Salvage and other sceptics were proved right.

Nurse tutors soon realised they would have to become even more skilled in the art of manipulating figures to meet their needs. Colleges were regularly under or over estimating how much it would cost to get the new style diploma programmes off the ground.

Department of Health officials were in despair as both sides realised the funding system was so hopelessly complicated that even if colleges had estimated their costs correctly, the information on which it was based could well be out of date by the time the courses were approved.

The transfer of education funds from the National Board to Regional Health Authorities in England only added to the confusion. Further anxiety and disappointment was created when RHAs decided that generally only one college per region should get the go-ahead to run courses in the first instance. Colleges claimed this had not been made clear to them and in several cases more than one institution per region had drawn up plans (*Nursing Times*, 1990a).

Many observers had warned that phased implementation of the reforms would have a deleterious impact, not only on the morale of educationalists, but on recruitment to the profession as a whole. Maude Storey, then RCN president, and not given to making alarmist statements, told RCN council; 'I am becoming more and more convinced of a political conspiracy' (*Nursing Times*, 1990a).

Her fears had been fuelled by the announcement only two weeks earlier of a delay in implementing Project 2000 in Wales, for 'resource reasons'. This created a storm of protest and culminated in RCN activists leading a delegation to the Welsh office. Senior figures, not familiar with placard waving denounced the delay, wrote to newspapers and lobbied MPs. The Welsh office eventually caved in. With support for the Conservative Party in Wales a worry for party strategists, could ministers afford to offend another group of potential supporters at the next general election?

Obviously the publicity was too much to bear. 'Everybody in Wales has campaigned hard for this, from the RCN to nurse tutors and MPs. We have had the support of both Labour MPs and Conservative backbenchers', said Anne Pegington, secretary of the RCN Welsh board (*Nursing Times*, 1990b).

Students started the new courses in England in the autumn of 1989, without a great deal of pomp and ceremony. In the first 18 months there was a great reluctance to talk publicly about any teething problems or wastage rates. But the students' attention was very much focused on the fact that their bursaries had been frozen at the 1989 level. The anger over this reached fever pitch in Spring 1991 as students campaigned for the bursary to be linked to the pay of other student nurses. But more senior nursing leaders wished the students would shut up and go back to their books! They feared the link with salaries would sully the waters and undermine the principle that students have supernumerary status.

The campaign saw NUPE, COHSE the RCN and NALGO student activists join forces around the country. Once again MPs were lobbied, letters written to local papers and petitions were circulated. The issue made good copy for reporters. The bursary freeze was the quintessential nursing hard luck story of the day as journalists had tired of recounting the depressing tale of clinical grading appeals. Tory MPs in marginal constituencies were also asking 'Why no increase?'.

The then Secretary of State for Health, William Waldegrave once again used RCN Congress to hand out prizes. The bursary would be increased on a one off basis, he told the audience, some of whom were ready to stage a publicity stunt if he had come to Harrogate with nothing. The argument for bursary levels to be tied in with Pay Review Body recommendations continues.

The quick response of the Welsh educationalists and the Project 2000 students, are good examples of how disagreeable ministerial decisions or inaction need more than just discreet letter writing and phone calls to civil servants. Making a noise wins rewards, but it has to be done with a bit of imagination and sophistication.

Relying on nursing statutory bodies during times such as these is of limited use. Although the Welsh National Board for Nursing, Midwifery and Health Visiting spoke out about the Project 2000 delay, the United Kingdom Central Council for Nursing, Midwifery and Health Visiting (UKCC) tempered its response.

Naturally with the monumental change Project 2000 brought, there were bound to be problems. But all those involved knew the ground would have to be laid carefully, so why then were some of the potential obstacles to smooth implementation, namely funding, inadvertently caused by government policy itself? Why did the Department of Health wait until February 1991 to send out an information pack to health authorities on Project 2000 when students had started in 1989? Virginia Bottomley, then health minister, tried to calm fears with statements in parliament expounding the virtues of Project 2000. 'Additional funding will be made available in future years against a background of other competing needs', she told MPs (*Nursing Times*, 1990c).

Fortunately with 1991 being a potential election year, Project 2000 did receive an extra boost, in the form of £98 million for 1992–93. This compared favourably with the year before, when it got £71 million (Department of Health, 1992). Nevertheless, resourcing the reforms still caused concern among teachers, not only in terms of cash, but library facilities, classroom space and teaching staff (Jowett et al., 1991) (Payne et al., 1991). The commitment of most civil servants to Project 2000 at the Department is not questioned, but the nature of the annual public expenditure bids will mean that it must be seen to be effective.

A closer look at some of the principles behind Project 2000 reveal it is the black sheep of the government's family of education reforms. Former Education Secretary Kenneth Clarke, a man well known to nurses for his years at the DoH, has told countless audiences that he wants to stamp out 'damaging 60s teaching styles' in centres of higher education.

Although Project 2000 is not necessarily going to be taught in that spirit, it is worth reflecting on what Mr Clarke said the day he announced changes to secondary teachers, training. 'Theory can be no substitute for this practical training in professions that give person to person services' (*Times Educational Supplement*, 1992; p7). Isn't it just a little odd that while nurse tutors are busy drawing up more academically rigorous courses for the practitioner of the future to create a 'knowledgeable doer' who will question the status quo, the government is intent on revamping the way secondary school teachers are trained?

Given this sort of ideology, it will only be a matter of time before Project 2000 is modified here and there, bit by bit. How can the emphasis on patient/client advocacy and encouraging critical thinking in Project 2000 curricula fit into the new style health service, where in some NHS Trusts it is a breach of contract to talk about your work to an outsider?

Tutors in the National Foundation for Educational Project 2000 Research (NFER) report feared that students who were heavily influenced by old fashioned ward cultures would threaten the creation of the critical thinker. So far few have dared criticise the reforms outright. Those inside the profession do not want to give critics of the reforms any ammunition. Those outside the profession who mutter disapproval speak for a powerful minority who are showing signs of working to undermine it, either by starving colleges of resources or claiming that the education of the nursing workforce does not fit into the manpower requirements of the future.

Surely it does not suit any government who wants a compliant workforce to have a new breed of nurse demanding more resources for health care, probing doctors and managers, and able to cogently use research to argue their case. As the former NHS personnel director Eric Caines said in an off-the-cuff but nevertheless revealing remark, 'Project 2000 students are going to see themselves as a pretty rarefied breed. Who is going to do the bread and butter work?' (*Nursing Times*, 1992)

Health care support workers – roles and relationships

The answer to Mr Caines question has to be the health care support worker (HCSW), the generic worker who will gain skills through National Vocational Qualifications. This group has had to endure so many title changes that it must be suffering an acute identity crisis by now. The fact that the term 'an army of support workers' has been coined indicates that nurses see them as a threat; they believe HCSWs will snatch bedside nursing away from qualified staff. There was a great stir in 1991 when it was suggested that HCSWs could look after patients with naso-gastric tubes, catheters, and tracheostomies. What some qualified staff have failed to grasp is that nursing auxiliaries have been doing much of this work for years and that National Vocational Qualifications (NVQs) offer them the opportunity to get training and recognition. They will also fill some of the gaps left by salaried student nurses.

Obviously it is essential that the new breed of assistants are competent and that they are accountable to nurses. In the main, they are likely to be, but only if nurses play an active part in discussions with the Care Sector Consortium and the NHS Training Directorate. It is not possible in this chapter to explore the full impact that HCSWs will have on nursing and midwifery, but trade unions have got their eyes keenly fixed on this group of potential new recruits.

The debate within the RCN as to whether to allow HCSWs into College membership is fascinating for what it reveals about qualified nurses' attitudes to those it classifies as 'unqualified.' The divide between those who welcome them with open arms and those who feel it will dilute professionalism within the world's largest nursing organisation is stark. Officially the College believes it is a good move to allow membership, a benevolent act that will only benefit both sides, as HCSWs will have access to a wide range of professional benefits. But it also wants control of this body of workers, and wants to define the lines of accountability. With the drop in qualified staff predicted for the next century, the tranche from additional members will be needed if the current growth in services is to be maintained.

Not surprisingly the new public sector union UNISON believes it is the natural union for HCSWs. Indeed the expected health service membership of this union will top or at least nudge the RCN's membership, but this will partly depend on how the formation of NHS trusts affects union representation and membership.

Remuneration: the problem that won't go away

With nurses pay accounting for £3 of every £100 of public expenditure (Clay, 1991), it is plain to see why controlling it has been the obsession of successive governments and personnel experts. Behind all the rhetoric about how nurses' and midwives' pay has increased by over 20% in the last ten years and an average of 17.9% in 1988 alone, at a cost of nearly £1 billion, there is a constant battle to keep pay to the absolute minimum necessary to recruit staff. The Conservative government believes regional pay and local pay is the way to do this, an approach fiercely resisted by unions.

The Pay Review Body has also cautioned against some of the more outrageous proposals for breaking up national pay bargaining. What is feared is nurses being paid the market rate, which would be higher in the South East of England and in some other metropolitan areas, but low in Northern England, Scotland, Wales and Northern Ireland and in areas blighted by high unemployment.

Regional pay variations, however, existed before the historic clinical grading agreement, with London weighting. Clinical grading was hailed as the panacea to the perennial recruitment and retention problem. It was supposed to be a national award, but its misapplication was due to the fact that such a huge organisational task had to be completed within a tight deadline.

The inequalities and distortions created by grading were in part a reflection of the government's desire to see regional pay slip in through the back door and its failure, yet again, to understand the complex nature of nursing and midwifery. The new pay structure raised a whole host of contentious professional issues. It revealed that thousands of nurses were doing jobs that they were not trained for, working unsupervised and taking on enormous amounts of responsibility. Above all, it revealed that all this unrecognised work was too expensive to pay for.

Research by the Institute of Manpower Studies has since shown nurses who do unpaid overtime and work through meal breaks are saving the NHS £567 million (Buchan, 1991). A massive 135, 000 NHS nursing and midwifery staff appealed against their grades; nearly a quarter of the nursing workforce (Gaze, 1990). There was widespread industrial action, with 'working to grade', where staff did not take on any duties they were not paid for. Ironically, the appeals outstanding against grades handed out in 1988 are still clogged in the system, and the cost of handling those appeals is probably more than what it would have cost to award the right grades in the first place.

The National Audit Office (the quango responsible for looking at value for money in government departments) has examined the cost to the health service of the grading appeals. Its findings are no doubt highly embarrassing for the government, but they will not be published as the NAO has not been asked to launch a full-scale enquiry into grading. Pay rates for the same job differ widely between districts, as MP for Liverpool Mossley Hill, David Alton, told the House of Commons.

Why has one staff midwife in ten in England and Wales been placed on scale D, but only one in 500 in Scotland? Why have half the staff midwives in Wales been placed on Scale F, but only one in eight in England? Why have 25% of midwifery sisters in Scotland and England been placed on scale F, but only 8% in Wales?

(Hansard, 1988)

The government denied any inconsistency and David Mellor, then health minister described the grading exercise as giving the profession 'the greatest shot in the arm it had ever had' (Hansard, 1988). Later on, the then secretary of state for health Kenneth Clarke said the NHS had made a 'horlicks' of clinical grading (*Nursing Times*, 1990d).

There were promises that grades would be awarded fairly, with management guidance to assist personnel officers. But this was twisted and used to alter skill mix, marginalise staff who did not 'fit in' (particularly black and ethnic minority nurses, enrolled nurses, and midwives) and down-grade staff who deserved and were promised higher pay. After all, at the back of everyone's minds was the need to control the workforce and stay within budget.

Nurses' pay has certainly increased, indeed some individuals did very well out of clinical grading. However, the pressures on staff have multiplied and they are still left wondering 'Are nurses now well paid?' The answer to that will depend on who you talk to. The government most certainly believes nurses are well paid. The RCN refrains from portraying nurses as low paid, because it detracts from their agenda of promoting nursing as a highly skilled profession.

A briefing supplied to journalists by the college says 'Most people assume nursing is a poorly paid profession, but two years ago a proper clinical grading structure was introduced, which aimed to reward nurses for work at the bedside' (Royal College of Nursing, 1990b). But it goes on to admit that staging the pay awards has meant nurses' pay has not kept up with inflation. This calculated move on the part of the government is saving millions, but is eroding the gains made in 1988.

It is not in any union leader's interest to admit that all nurses' pay is poor, or that the grading exercise was a catastrophe, as it only reflects badly on them as negotiators. But the fact is that nurses on the lower grades, who do not qualify for supplements and London allowances, still earn a meagre wage considering the responsibility they take on and the stress endured. Enrolled nurses still earn less than the average female wage (Appleby and Brewins, 1992). A grade E staff nurse working in a busy Accident and Emergency department outside London could in November 1991 hope for £13, 000 a year at the most.

Many people have asked why the unions agreed to clinical grading being implemented within such a short timetable and without the option of top up funds if necessary. Did they fear that without seizing the opportunity, the offer of a new pay spine would vanish into thin air?

Whatever the reason, they accepted the new pay spine, which in most people's view was the right decision, but the wounds it inflicted took a long time to heal and those who found themselves inadequately rewarded are still bearing the scars.

Industrial action versus creative protest

The industrial action that rocked the NHS in 1988 was not born exclusively out of anger at the threatened withdrawal of special duty payments and clinical grading. Emotions had been running high from the previous year when the perpetual financial crisis in the NHS reached new depths. RCN members were balloted on whether they wanted to retain Rule 12, which prevents industrial action, and after a debate about the bias in the wording of the ballot, the no-strike policy was kept. The Royal College of Midwives followed suit. Despite both college's decisions, some of their members did take industrial action, which demonstrates that in some circumstances it can be the only sanction left, and that it still has a role.

Some people argue that nurses, like other employees have the right to withdraw their labour. Indeed doctors in Britain have threatened to strike at least twice in the early 1990s. Often it is only the threat of industrial action that has the desired effect. Those that accuse strikers in the caring professions of being irresponsible should remember that no nurse ever uses the sanction without very careful consideration.

It seems that Trevor Clay in 'Nurses, Power and Politics', believes it is only British nurses who have a 'pact with the public'. They have worked hard to earn respect over many years; nurses are not automatically adored by the public, he argues (Clay, 1987).

Obviously at the time of writing this he could not have predicted the outcome of big disputes in Canada, Australia, New Zealand, France and elsewhere. Although the strikers have had mixed success in winning all their demands, public opinion was on their side.

On the Australian dispute in 1986–7, in the Southern state of Victoria, the *British Medical Journal* reported 'The really surprising thing about the dispute was the support that nurses got' (Knight, 1987). The journal later noted 'The strike lasting 50 days led to the government conceding almost everything that the Royal Australian Nursing Federation (the union) had been requesting for months before the strike' (Delamothe, 1988). French nurses struck in 1988 and again in 1991 over pay and conditions. They are split between two unions which does not help to present a united front. This however, did not stop them from staging sit-ins, and as a result having water cannon and tear gas fired on them. The French nurses action had the backing of the public. Seventy-eight per cent of those questioned in a poll believed nurses were right to strike (Snell, 1991). Public support for all out strike action can quickly dwindle and it is easy to understand why the RCN opposes this. However, it is part of the culture of TUC activists to call for demonstrations, and to visibly protest, whereas the RCN approach is to work behind the scenes. As typified in the campaign against the introduction of general managers, there is a reliance on high profile advertising. Writing letters to politicians and expressing concern through high level committees are other favoured techniques. But some of these methods by-pass lay voters, the users of the service, the people whose support could add weight to any campaign.

An RCN committee set up in 1979 to explore alternative 'professional' forms of action decided that there was nothing nurses could do that would not threaten the 'pact with the public'. The decision displayed a remarkable lack of imagination. Sit-ins, demonstrations with an unusual theme, pickets, wearing civilian clothing to work, donning black arm bands and other stunts do not have to harm patients and clients. (Bed pushes used to be a popular form of protest, but now seem to have gone out of fashion.) These sort of actions can do a lot to reduce frustration and powerlessness and inject team spirit, thus raising morale.

The RCN would frown upon the approach of French nurses who wore hospital gowns, oxygen masks, and face masks in spectacular street demonstrations; these were nevertheless visually powerful images and succeeded in alerting the government, through the media, to the fact that nurses were 'at the end of their tether', (Snell, 1991).

Although action by policy-makers may not be immediate, the potency of such images and the degree to which they stick in peoples' minds, should not be underestimated.

Media image – fact or fiction

When BBC radio health correspondent Niall Dickson was compiling a progress report on the NHS reforms in January 1992, the RCN press office had to speak to ten district nurses before one was willing to be interviewed on the 'Today' news and current affairs programme. Doctors and managers were willing to speak and were articulate and confident that their position of authority would see them through any tussle with senior colleagues.

His experience is typical of many journalists trying to cover a nursing story. Even when nurses are the natural experts on a particular subject, or key witnesses to gross injustice, they are reluctant to speak to the media. Part of this apparent unwillingness is due to a lack of confidence and understanding of the way the media works.

It is also an industrial relations issue as many nurses' employment contracts prohibit disclosure of work-related activities to the media without permission. But it is also a reflection of nurses undervaluing their knowledge and believing that essentially male doctors and managers are better equipped to impart information. This is also the case in other public arenas. It is no coincidence that many of the nurses who ask questions at conferences attended mainly by women, are men (see Chapters 1 and 3).

Men are more likely to be outspoken branch secretaries of unions and will speak to the press more freely than many women do. How many nurse columnists are there in national newspapers? There were at least three doctor columnists at the time of writing.

It seems that although nurses are held in high esteem by the public, they obviously do not yet command enough 'expertise' in the eyes of newspaper editors to warrant having a platform. Clare Raynor is a much celebrated nurse and agony aunt, but it was not primarily as a professional nurse that she was employed to give advice.

In 1991, the Department of Health medical advisors got themselves into a state of confusion over whether or not women should regularly perform breast self-examination. Contradictory information was given, undoing the hard work of those who had been for years persuading women to check their breasts monthly.

It was the medics and politicians, however, who tried to set the record straight. Despite the fact that there are hundreds of breast care nursing specialists in the UK and a woman chief nurse at the Department of Health, it was these two groups who did not feel constrained to pass judgement!

This was already a public relations disaster for the Department of Health. Surely it would have been better to have had a woman professional go on television to explain the importance of breast self-examination. A nurse would have been very well placed to reassure the worried female population about early treatment of a disease that still kills more women in the UK than nearly anywhere else in the Western world.

To cite another example, why was there not a huge profile in a national newspaper of England's new chief nursing officer (CNO) Yvonne Moores when she took office? Sir Kenneth Calman, the chief medical officer (CMO) was given an extensive write-up in *The Guardian* newspaper (Dean, 1991). He, like Mrs Moores is a civil servant, but it seems the CMO is much more likely to be pushed into the media limelight than the CNO. Why should this be? It is certainly no reflection on her considerable expertise and the public persona she presents.

The RCN is acutely aware of the need to promote professional and political issues in nursing, and has a well-resourced external affairs division. Despite this trend, nursing statutory bodies, (with the exception of a few proactive people inside them) have remained singularly unaware of the practicalities of press deadlines and the principles of news gathering. The fact that they have seemingly not bothered to develop a coherent public relations strategy bears this out. Localised newly formed specialist groups who do not have media-awareness training still tend to shy away from sustained high profile activity. A good example of this was when the Amalgamated School Nurses Association (ASNA) launched a campaign and report to save school nurses from extinction in January 1992 (Fletcher and Balding, 1992). Health authority cuts and the failure of policy makers to recognise the work of school nurses was threatening the speciality, the association said. But at the press conference, the school nurses (flanked by doctors) took a back seat when faced with questioning journalists.

The doctors, who endorsed the report, ended up being the school nurses' advocates and issuing stronger pleas on their behalf to the waiting media. During the photocall, the doctor (who it has to be said did a good job in raising the school nurses' profile), was the centre of attention. He stood holding the ASNA report while they looked on admiringly!

Nurses have to take control (and that means not allowing photographers and reporters to dictate the agenda during an interview) and learn to use the media to their own ends. Publicity can be an immensely powerful and positive tool to promote a cause among colleagues and more importantly, the users of the service. When this happens their image will shift further away from that of being the doctors' handmaiden to the autonomous professional who can offer succour and authoritative advice.

> It is not that nurses do not speak; reticence comes about because what they have to say is not valued by those in power and is not listened to . . .

Ward sisters and charge nurses represent the epitome of interface between management, located as they are at the intersection of a whole range of competing demands, interconnecting work relationships, overlapping professional boundaries, occupational groups and agencies. They stand at the meeting point of hospital and community, patient and relatives.

(Hart, 1991)

Who better than nurses to trumpet the message to the wider world?

NHS reforms: order or chaos?

By the time RCN general secretary Christine Hancock took office in September 1989, it was already too late to hold back the reforms, though she quickly identified the quality issue and the prospects for a pilot scheme which saw light the following spring in the House of Lords with the launch of the joint Royal Colleges' initiative.

Her predecessor, Trevor Clay, had achieved apparent victories with Project 2000 and clinical grading, and it was not yet apparent that Project 2000 would be in any way problematical or that a mistake had been made in allowing clinical grading to be cash limited.

There were complaints from members of all nursing unions in 1988, and there was a perceived lack of leadership about why the NHS reforms were such a bad thing. A discussion on the findings of a Consumer Connection report (unpublished, 1989) on RCN members attitudes to the NHS reforms was delayed while Trevor Clay and other leaders were at the International Council of Nurses meeting in South Korea, and several critical campaigning months were lost. Through that autumn RCN members were encouraged to send postcards to their MPs on the theme of a two-tier health service, and the party conferences were lobbied on that point.

However, any prospect for a joint campaign with other unions was beset with disagreement; the BMA chose to go it alone much of the time, and a joint effort on Trusts, a campaigning pack on the verge of publication, never appeared due to BMA hesitation. Perhaps it is true that the oft-repeated claim of constant reorganisation had left people tired. And perhaps the cooperation on the TUC demonstration in March 1988 opposing Prime Minister Margaret Thatcher's NHS review was as much joint action as could be mustered. Some trade union activists were even prepared to admit that trust status may have been the only way mental health and mental handicap units could secure extra or ring-fenced resources, a view shared by some community nurses (Tattam, 1991a).

Whilst it may be true that some of the wilder schemes proposed by the Adam Smith Institute, including health care vouchers, may have been dramatically altered or indeed dropped as a result of professional protest, it is clear that even in the face of public concern, the Government, with its large parliamentary majority, did not feel compelled to consult anyone, even the doctors. They, along with the trade unions, almost completely gave up the fight once it became clear that by the end of the century nearly every hospital would be a Trust and a large proportion of GP practices would become fundholding.

No matter how carefully the relationship had been cultivated at the top between ministers and professional leaders, without widespread grassroots revolt and a consistent message delivered to MPs at local level there was no altering the ideological course of the reforms. The culture of Scotland and Wales meant that at first they were left largely untouched, at least in terms of initial trust bids.

There was a small victory in the Clinical Standards Advisory Group. However, according to the government the real cure for the ills of the health service lay in the Patient's Charter, which has always been portrayed as a personal crusade by the Prime Minister, John Major. The Patient's Charter, has of course introduced the concept of the 'named nurse'. Being optimistic, some people in the profession thought this represented an extension of primary nursing. There is no doubt the 'named nurse initiative' could provide the opportunity for visionaries to personalise care. However, given the other demands of the Patient's Charter, it would seem in some instances it is likely to remain a public relations exercise, swamped by the overwhelming need to cut waiting lists and survive in the internal market.

In the 1992 general election campaign, like pressure groups and other trade unions, nursing had to stand on the sidelines while the politicians shamelessly exploited the health issue with accusations of horrific waiting lists on one hand, and scaremongering on the other. In actual fact, health, perceived as a vote winner for Labour, was effectively neutralised by the Conservatives as the major parties traded insults.

What these things illustrate is that politics is with us every day. Nurses at the highest level and at local level have got to take risks and speak out, pushing the Patient's Charter to its limits. Then, when the next proposals for change come along, a more articulate, informed, and individually assertive workforce will have laid the groundwork. Too much nursing energy is directed internally. For this to change, nurses need to feel at ease in public life, by, for example, writing letters to the local and national press (not just the nursing press) and appearing on radio and television. Professions do not have political clout until they become regular players in political life.

GNC to UKCC – a break with the past?

In its relatively short life, the UK supreme governing body for nurses, midwives and health visitors has created a bureaucracy and a culture that is more fitting for an organisation growing up in the 1950s. Although its work to promote reforms in nursing education is certainly an achievement and the Code of Conduct has done more to remind practitioners of their obligations to patients and clients than anything else in recent years, the council remains relatively remote and inaccessible to the people for whom it exists. The numerous committees of the UKCC seem bogged down in the minutiae of protocol and even the most uncontroversial matters are debated in closed sessions. Important information on the plans for post registration education were discussed in closed session, so that when the press and public had the 'information package' presented to them, there was no real opportunity for questions or debate at that time. Draft proposals for the future of community nursing education were drawn up in secret meetings. Although the professions had been consulted on these proposals, to observers at the UKCC's meetings, major decisions seem go through 'on the nod'. Members often seem reluctant to probe council officers views.

The decision to purchase a mews house, for the use of UKCC members, was made in a closed session of its finance committee. This was done to invest surplus funds. A UKCC employee, who wished to remain anonymous, also claimed 18 months earlier that there were staff shortages and that the professions were not getting a good service from the UKCC. This gives the impression the money spent on the mews house could have been put to better use. 'The UKCC is trying to administer nurses in this country as cheaply as possible', he said. The failure of the UKCC to publish election results also caused a row (*Nursing Standard*, 1989).

All this did not go unnoticed by Peat Marwick McLintock, the accountancy firm called in to examine the nursing Statutory Bodies. It produced a damning report of the UKCC's work (Peat Marwick McClintock, 1989. Legislation is now in place to reform the Statutory Bodies, which will become leaner outfits. The council is now functioning as an entirely elected body. But whether this will engender a greater need for public debate about policy in open meetings remains to be seen. While nurses fear the power the UKCC has to strike them off the register, this reverence is also tinged with hostility. The introduction of the periodic registration fee (which spelled an end to newly qualified staff getting the old General Nursing Council badge and traditional certificate in 1983) meant this big new ruling body did not immediately command the respect it wanted among practitioners.

The UKCC received hundreds of protest letters and was even taken to the High Court over periodic registration (it won the case). But one protest that revealed the depth of anger towards the fee was the delivery to the UKCC of a bag of blood, to symbolise 'getting blood out of a stone'. The practitioner in question is understood to have received a warning that this act of black humour could in itself have breached the code of conduct. Periodic registration fees were the price the profession had to pay to have a self-financing regulatory body. Nowadays most people consider it a price worth paying to remain semi-independent of government. But all the statutory bodies are governed by legislation which many complain limits their powers. Indeed the Peat Marwick McLintock report claimed their roles were blurred by unclear laws.

This is evident when one discovers the inability of the UKCC to pass on detailed information it has about poor standards of care in a particular authority or institution in the independent sector to the relevant agencies.

The process of investigating cases of misconduct can uncover a wealth of information about a particular institution, and on a number of occasions can point to serious mismanagement and other maltreatment of patients/clients. It is not the role of the UKCC to launch major investigations; all it can do is prove or disprove misconduct under the code, suspend a practitioner for a period of time from the register, or refer individuals for help.

UKCC members have expressed a great deal of frustation about knowing which are the 'blackspots', but the council has no formal way of passing the information it has gathered to, for example the Health Advisory Service, the Mental Health Act Commission, or the Clinical Standards Advisory Group. However, it can send transcripts of cases to Regional Health Authorities to alert them to areas of concern. As the UKCC is charged with protecting and improving standards of care, it is staggering that there is not enough flexibility in the legislation to allow an exchange of information. When the council sought legal advice it was told it could not extend its role to this area.

The code of conduct itself has the potential to be enormously powerful. It makes it mandatory for nurses to report poor standards, and those that do not can themselves be found guilty of misconduct. But it puts practitioners in a double bind. Many have tried to use it to improve standards of care in the workplace, but have found themselves dubbed trouble makers, victimised, or worse, lost their jobs. Graham Pink, the campaigning nurse from Stockport, Greater Manchester, who blew the whistle on poor standards of care in elderly care wards, continually cited the code, but was eventually dismissed from his post as charge nurse. Pink has frequently said the Code of Conduct ought to be carried with a health warning (Turner, 1992). Others are also concerned:

'The problem is the UKCC has . . . no authority at local level. It can offer advice and fine words but it has no mechanism with which to offer constructive support when the trouble starts', says Peter Fox, chair of the RCN Association for the Care of the Elderly. (Turner 1991)

The RCN was urged by its members to campaign for a stronger code, but it seems this has not been done with any of the vigour needed to affect change in an organisation like the UKCC. In recognition of the fact that the UKCC code did not afford enough protection to questioning practitioners, the college set up its own whistleblowing service, which allowed people to write and inform RCN officers of bad practice. The informants are protected and the local officers take up the case discreetly with managers. As the RCN is retaining the confidentiality of whistleblowers, it is difficult to know whether it has been truly able to rectify problem situations. It could be that it just serves to make the informant feel better for having 'done something'. It is hoped the approaches made by RCN representatives to local managers are enough to make them look at staffing levels, or any other factors that may be the root cause of the problem.

The revised code contains a number of improvements, but does not contain any panacea for whistleblowers. Practitioners still only have an obligation to inform someone of circumstances which may jeopardise standards of care. Hence legislation is called for to protect those brave enough to question managers. (Tattam, 1991b). This has not been forthcoming; however Health Secretary Virginia Bottomley launched an appeals system for those wishing to complain about standards, demonstrating that cases like Graham Pink's have not gone unnoticed in Whitehall. Ironically, one of the first critics of Mrs Bottomley's guidance was the chief executive of Stockport Health Authority, who claimed that the sort of guidance recommended was in place when Mr Pink made his claims about standards of care.

On Being a Political Nurse

Being political these days is not just about knowing who the health minister is and who controls the purse strings of health care. It is more than writing to your MP. It is about understanding the significance and the effect that national, regional, and local power structures have on nurses as employees and professionals. An interest in politics and decision making is not created overnight; it is an evolutionary process that is spurred on usually by personal and financial grievance or the ongoing desire to see change.

However, it does not always have to be the natural result of negative experiences. Being educated to accept accountability is part of the process of becoming political. The provision of health care and nurses as the main providers of care, has been high on the political agenda, and will continue to be with nursing consuming 40% of the £30 billion spent on the NHS (Clay, 1991). Any political party that ignores it does so at its peril. However when ministers wax lyrical about the importance of nurses and how the government values their hard work, are they at the same time ready and willing to listen to their fears, concerns and visions for the future? Any government will appear to listen until such time as the message becomes unpalatable or the vision defies its already clearly mapped out agenda.

So is there a firm political agenda for nursing and for health care and is it what it seems? It was certainly not in the Conservative Party's 1987 election manifesto; and despite the emerging shape of the future NHS, as enshrined in the NHS and Community Care Act 1990, if you were to ask members of the cabinet what their agenda was for health care for the remainder of the century, they probably would give you the answer you might expect. The NHS should be offering a better quality of care and more choice to patients within a cost efficient health care system. This really does not say much and it might as easily be British Rail they are talking about!

According to opposition politicians, the Conservative Party wants to privatise the NHS 'through the back door'. The 'creeping commercialisation of care' demonstrates what they say. If we look at that statement in 20 years time, it will probably have been a more or less accurate prediction, but one that at the moment seems like just another slogan in the war of words fought over the NHS.

Politicians use the NHS and nurses as the caring face of the service, to score political points but few of them are able to grasp its complexities. Their version of events and plans for the future are recounted in television interviews and debates in parliament. However, stories often bear no resemblance to the reality on the ground. For example, David Mellor, then health minister, praised the Department of Health's Strategy for Nursing for being a 'world first' when he addressed a conference at the King's Fund Centre in June 1989:

'The future of nursing in this country seems to be bright and full of promise', he said. The great and the good had been meeting to talk about how the strategy could be translated into action – no mean feat. At the time, the *Nursing Times* noted that although the production of any sort of document at all was an achievement, 'there were no teeth behind it to ensure it was implemented. Perhaps the best the profession can hope for is that in repeating what it wants loud and long enough someone will listen' (Snell, 1989). To many people, that 'someone' was William Waldegrave, the man who added the gentle touch to the DOH after the departure of Kenneth Clarke to Education and the ousting of Margaret Thatcher as Prime Minister.

Under Clarke, the chief nurse Anne Poole was denied a place on the NHS policy board, an omission Waldegrave rectified within months of becoming Secretary of State. This and an injection of millions of pounds for nursing developments gave the profession, still recovering from the shock of the clinical grading exercise and a perceived attack on its middle management structure, a much needed boost.

William Waldegrave seemed genuinely interested in nursing, so much so that whoever met him on visits to nursing development units were bowled over by his enthusiasm. They had never seen it before in a politician, yet he was replaced after the 1992 General Election by Virginia Bottomley. It is important to remember that in politics, it is the present that counts above all else. Nurses have had to learn this the hard way.

The need for accountability is recognised in a practitioner's professional life, but why shouldn't this attitude extend into political activism in society at large? To be seen to care and yet to challenge politically both inside and outside the workplace, may seem to be a challenging, overt agenda. In reality it offers a great opportunity for professional and personal growth, which can only improve the care given to patients and clients far more profoundly than the covert methods of the past. As Marie Manthey, president of the Creative Nursing Management company, Minneapolis and founder of primary nursing in the United States says: 'Anyone who experiences a problem enough to talk about it, owns it and has both the right and the responsibility to participate in solving it' (Davidson, 1992).

References

Alderman, P. (1991). The other lady of the Crimea. *The Lady*, **214 (SSS)** 1238.

Appleby, J. and Brewins, L. (1992). Profile of a profession. *Nursing Times*, **88(4)**, 24–7.

Audit Commission (1991). *The Virtue of Patients*: *Making Best Use of Ward Nursing Resources*. HMSO, London.

Buchan, J. (1991). *Nurses' Work and Worth*: *Pay, Careers and Working Patterns of Qualified Nurses*. (IMS Report 213). Institute of Manpower Studies, Falmer.

Clay, T. (1987). *Nurses*: *Power and Politics*. Heinemann, London.

Clay, T. (1989). Nursing and politics: The unquiet relationship. In *Current Issues in Nursing*, M. Jolley and P. Allan (eds), Chapman & Hall, London, pp. 115–29.

Clay, T. (1991). *Nursing into the 1990s*. King Edward's Hospital Fund, London.

Davidson, L. (1992). Morale imperative. *Nursing Times*, **88(23)**, 20–1.

Dean, M. (1991) Monday profile: healthy streak of subversion. *The Guardian* 14 October, 23.

Delamothe, T. (1988). Nurses: where do they go from here? *British Medical Journal*, **296(6620)**, 449.

Department of Health (1992). *£98m injection for pioneering nurse education scheme*. Department of Health, London. (Press Release H92/12).

Fletcher, K. and Balding, J. (1992). *School Nurses Do It in Schools: Trends in School Nursing Practice*. Amalgamated School Nurses Association, Huntingdon.

Gaze, H. (1990). The forgotten fifty thousand. *Nursing Times*, **86(6)**, 28–31.

Hansard (1988). Midwives (grading review). *Hansard: House of Commons*, **143(13)**, cols 407–16.

Hancock, C. (1991). Speech to membership groups. (Unpublished.)

Hart, E. (1991). Ghost in the machine. *Health Service Journal*, **101(5281)**, 20–2.

Havel, V. (1989). *Vaclav Havel: or Living in Truth*. Faber, London.

Jowett, S., Walton, I. and Payne, S. (1991). *The NFER Project 2000 Research: an Introduction and Some Interim Issues*. (Interim paper 2.) National Foundation for Educational Research, Slough.

Kinnock, N. (1985). Speech to Labour Party Conference. (Unpublished.)

Knight, J. (1987). Victorian nurses' strike. *British Medical Journal*, **294(6568)**, 363–4.

Lee-Cunin, M. (1989). *Daughters of Seacole: a Study of Black Nurses in West Yorkshire*. West Yorkshire Pay Unit, Batley.

Nursing Standard (1989). UKCC election row. *Nursing Standard*, **3(16)**, 6.

Nursing Times (1990a). Anger over 'broken promises' on P2000. *Nursing Times*, **86(21)**, 5.

Nursing Times (1990b). Welsh Office backs down. *Nursing Times*, **86(29)**, 7.

Nursing Times (1990c). Minister pledges P2000 funds will continue. *Nursing Times*, **86(28)**, 5

Nursing Times (1990d). Quotes. *Nursing Times*, **86(1)**, 20.

Nursing Times (1992). Quotes of the year. *Nursing Times*, **88(1)**, 15.

Payne, S., Jowett, S. and Walton, I. (1991). *Nurse Teachers in Project 2000: the Experience of Planning and Initial Implementation*. (Interim paper 3.) National Foundation for Educational Research, Slough.

Peat Marwick McLintock (1989). *Review of the United Kingdom Central Council and the Four National Boards for Nursing, Midwifery and Health Visiting*. Department of Health, London.

Royal College of Nursing (1989). Consumer Connection Report (Unpublished)

Royal College of Nursing (1990a). *Meeting the Challenge of Racial Equality in Nursing: a Discussion Document*. RCN, London.

Royal College of Nursing (1990b). Journalists' briefing: Department of External Affairs. (Unpublished.)

Salvage, J. (1985). *The Politics of Nursing*. Heinemann, London.

Salvage, J. (1988). Brighton Breezes. *Nursing Times*, **84(24)**, 22.

Snell, J. (1989). Planning the future. *Nursing Times*, **85(28)**, 22–3.

Snell, J. (1991). Les Miserables. *Nursing Times*, **87(45)**, 23.

Snell, J. (1992). Black nurses 'lost out' in clinical regrading. *Nursing Times*, **88(25)**, 6.

Spectator, (1988). Carry on, Nurse. *Spectator*, 28 May, 5.

Tattam, A. (1991a). Can we trust the trusts? *Nursing Times*, 87(39), 16–70.

Tattam, A. (1991b). Call for laws on whistle-blowing. *Nursing Times*, **87(50)**, 6.

Times Educational Supplement (1992). What the minister said. *Times Educational Supplement*, 10 January,7.

Turner, T. (1992). The indomitable Mr Pink. *Nursing Times*, **88(24)**, 26–9.

Turner, T. (1991). A paper tiger? *Nursing Times*, **87(24)**, 20.

6 Nursing values: nightmares and nonsense

It is fashionable these days to talk about the 'value of nursing', and much is being written concerning the development of and fostering of the right and presumably correct nursing values. But the central question must still remain – what are values? What do nurses mean when they talk about values and is it the same as what philosophers and ethicists mean? Can there be personal and professional values and need these always be congruent?

Definitions of 'values' in the context of moral philosophy vary, but most definitions contain an element of worthiness and personal appraisal – thus the *Shorter Oxford English Dictionary* defines 'value' as

> the relative status of a thing, or the estimate in which it is held according to its real or supposed worth, usefulness and importance . . . estimate of or liking of a person or thing . . . to consider of worth or importance; to rate high; to esteem, to set store by, to take account of, to heed or be concerned about, to care, to pride or plume oneself on or upon a thing, to think highly of oneself for something . . . one's principles or standards; one's judgement of what is valuable or important in life . . . (*Shorter Oxford English Dictionary*, 1973)

Some of these definitions will seem familiar enough, some will appear rather controversial; for example, a definition of 'value' which addresses the issue of care and caring, or the notion of self-valuing or even pride in identification. All these aspects of value, valuing and values are present in the English language, and as Kopelman (1984) points out 'language is a subtle indicator of social mores'.

Values are of particular importance to health care professionals because it is precisely how we think and feel about issues and aspects of life that ultimately governs our behaviour. It is because of the cognitive and affective aspects of valuing that philosophers and ethicists, not only nurses and other members of the health care professions, have interested themselves in various aspects of valuing and values clarification.

Although the roots of values clarification may be Eastern, or an American-ised (and sanitised) version of some mystical endeavour, values clarification, as accepted by the nursing profession, is an attempt to identify and literally clarify the nature of one's most powerful values (Inglesby, 1992). Of course, as Inglesby notes,

> For those who are secure either in their religious belief or cultural traditions, the need to question fundamental assumptions about life

and meaning does not exist. If the symbols of one's culture are mean-ingful they do not need exploration. It is only when they no longer match the feelings they are meant to represent that analysis appears necessary.

This chapter will look at some of the issues raised by moral philosophers and nursing leaders in regard to the nature of values and the need for values clarification, suggesting that the nursing profession espouses certain professional values that at best have outlived their usefulness, and by analysing the nature of nursing practice a better understanding of positive values will be achieved. We can only foster and encourage to flourish those values which we can identify, isolate and find worthy of our support; 'Ultimately, what is done is influenced by the values of the person initiating it. People do what they do largely because of what they value' (Ashworth, 1988).

The initial task is to determine the relationship between personal and professional values. All people value something, even the greatest exponent of egoism values something, presumably his own estimation of his self-worth. Early Greek philosophers such as Socrates and Aristotle were concerned with aspects of valuing because they understood the connection between prizing certain things, and behaving accordingly.

Socrates is represented as the archetypal mentor, whose role it was to constantly challenge his followers *to think* why they felt in a certain way, what was the source of their reasoning, what values were underpinning their thoughts, and thereby their actions. This form of intellectual stimulation is not always appreciated, as Plato often pointed out; the master's aim in this exercise was to show the connection between what we value, how we reason, and the subsequent effect this has on conscious (and unconscious) action, which leads to an analysis of the nature of virtue and it cultivation; that is, the cultivation of positive and prized actions.

Socrates, after a lengthy discussion with Meno, concluded that virtue consists of true opinion and knowledge, and that the 'possession of which makes a man a true guide . . . where human control leads to right ends, these two principles are directive, true opinion and knowledge' (Meno: 99a, in Hamilton and Cairns, 1961). However, no sooner does Socrates utter these words, than he hastens to correct and edit what he thinks, for he claims: 'Since virtue cannot be taught, we can no longer believe it to be knowledge, so that one of our two good and useful principles is excluded, and knowledge is not the guide in public life' (Meno: 99b, in Hamilton and Cairns, 1961). This observation is one of the central controversial aspects of any debate concerning the nature of values, human action and virtues, for there certainly is a large body of opinion which claims that since virtue cannot be taught, it is not part of knowledge (personal or collective), and therefore analysis of how and why we reason will not effectively alter our behaviour. The purpose of analysing one's values is not, according to these thinkers, in order to teach others similar patterns of reasoning, but in order to be more aware of that which governs our own private and public actions, for only such endeavours can promote an understanding of the nature of virtue. As Murdoch comments, these philosophers would say that 'we ought to know what we are doing' (Murdoch, 1970). Needless to say, not all philosophers see the nature of virtues and their underlying values in the same way.

Thompson and Thompson (1990) add that 'values are more often "caught" from than taught by a faculty. If you wish to understand your dominant nursing values, think back to the important faculty and preceptors in your basic education as well as those you consider your mentors in the profession today.'

Nagel (1980), in a treatise on 'The Limits of Objectivity' picks up the polemic, so unpopular with modern nurse theorists, on the nature of objectivity in relationship to value and values. If some things, endeavours, notions, and concerns, have *more* value than others, is this prizing and valuing always, of necessity, subjective, or can there be an element of objectivity in what we value? The answer to this problem is crucial for the nursing profession, which assumes, rather uniformly, that values 'are the "why's" that give us a sense of meaning and purpose in nursing' (Uustal, 1987). What is not clear at all, however, is how these values are arrived at, and whether or not nursing values represent subjective or objective values.

As Nagel notes 'whether values can be objective depends on whether an interpretation of objectivity can be found that allows us to advance our knowledge of what to do, what to want, and what things provide reasons for and against action' (Nagel, 1980). Nagel makes the point, initiated by Socrates, that 'values are neither physical nor mental' and therefore presumably notions of perceptions must be applied with caution, and in any event, he observes 'Not all values are likely to prove to be objective in any sense' (Nagel, 1980). This is important to remember, for although undoubtedly we may be able to define some values objectively, such as wealth or even health, others will always remain questionably subjective; as, for example, matters of taste in art or aspects of emotions; although even these values have been qualified and subjectively defined, especially matters of aesthetics (Aristotle, 1920).

Nagel contends that 'objectivity is advanced when we step back, detached from our earlier point of view toward something, and arrive at a new view of the whole that is formed by *including ourselves* and our earlier viewpoint in what is to be understood' (Nagel, 1980) (emphasis mine). It is important to note that in his definition of attempting to identify objectivity in relationship to values, he includes the deliberate use of self. We can only be objective about something that matters *to us*. Those matters that do not concern us, are not included in pursuit of value objectivity, they are agent-neutral matters, which is not the same thing.

Nagel proceeds to define objectivity to mean 'that when we detach from our individual perspective and the values and reasons that seem acceptable from within it, we can sometimes arrive at a new conception which may endorse some of the original reasons but will reject some as subjective appearances and add others. This values clarification exercise is probably quite familiar to nurses, as Nagel concludes, 'The basic step of placing ourselves and our attitudes within the world to be considered is familiar, but the form of the result – a new set of values, reason and motives – is different.'

Many nurses endorse exercises to encourage values identification and clarification, but with a totally subjective agenda, for in the words of Uustal

(1987), '*Your* values directly influence *your* ethical reasoning and choices on both conscious and unconscious levels' (emphasis mine). Examining values for their intrinsic worth is seen as an important process in the course of professionalisation, where 'Professional values come through socialisation in a career' (Thompson and Thompson, 1990). Since 'the price you pay for unexamined values is often confusion, indecision and inconsistency . . . the clearer you are about what you value, the more able you are to choose and initiate a response that is consistent with what you say you believe' (Uustal, 1987). This statement, however, does not of itself help us in deciding whether it is ever possible to have objective values, that is, values held in common by a group of like-minded people and reflected in similar philosophies and practice, as would be so in the instance of a profession. As Nagel comments:

> In order to discover whether there are any objective values or reasons we must try to arrive at *normative* judgements, with *motivational content*, from an impersonal standpoint, a standpoint outside of our lives. We cannot use a *non-normative* criterion of objectivity: for *if* any values are objective, they are objective *values*, not objective anything else.
>
> (Nagel, 1980)

Nurses often comment that theirs is a *practical* art and science, and that they perform best when allowed to marry knowledge with practice. Nagel (1980) states that 'practical objectivity means that practical reason can be understood and even engaged in by the objective self'.

The trick appears to be to acknowledge the existence of personal values objectively, since 'values are described as personal in nature and involving affective responses' (Uustal, 1987). However, because their existence is reflected in public, and not only private behaviour, they can be objectively assessed, or at least said to have objective components. Thus,

> We want to be able to understand and accept the way we live from outside, but it may not always follow that we should control our lives from inside by the terms of that external understanding. Often the objective viewpoint will not be suitable as a replacement for the subjective, but will co-exist with it, setting a standard with which the subjective is constrained not to clash.
>
> (Nagel, 1980)

Thompson and Thompson (1990) note that 'Self-knowledge, or awareness is an essential ingredient for fulfilling one's professional role as a nurse . . . To make ethical decisions in practice, one needs to know and understand both ethics and the personal and professional values that direct one's daily life.' In order to know and understand one's personal and professional values, it would appear that an ongoing process of values clarification needs to be instituted.

It is seen as insufficient to simply identify and clarify the values we profess. Part of the hidden agenda in regards to value clarification is the very admissibility of change and multiplicity of values. Thompson and Thompson (1990) state that 'values can be changed' quoting Massey who considers that 'values need to be consciously known in order to be evaluated and changed. Values change in response to *adult reasoning* instead of, or in addition to, emotional impacts' (emphasis mine). A sentiment shared no doubt by Socrates. James Rest, cited by Thompson and Thompson (1990) in comment on moral development, suggests in Kohlbergian terms (Kohlberg, 1969) a sequential approach to the change of values; namely, we recognise a value, then we understand it, come to prefer it, and finally practice it. This of course mirrors the three elements necessary in order for a value indicator to be considered a 'value'. Based on the original work of Raths *et al.* (1978), the process of valuing is seen to incorporate elements of freely choosing a value from alternatives, prizing the value that one chooses, and finally acting unconsciously on the bases of the free choice in public, and consistently (Uustal, 1987).

We would like to think that we always make conscious free choices concerning our values. However, as Thompson and Thompson (1990) point out, citing experts in the field, we are probably 'programmed with 90 percent of our personal (gut level) values by the age of 10, and the remaining 10 percent by the age of 20'. This does not bode well for mature nurses. No wonder nursing leaders are calling for a re-examination of our *personal* values, making Reilly (1989) somberly comment 'that most of us agree that nursing is a value-laden practice'. Reilly is quite emphatic in stating that 'value development through choice, rather than through fiat, is different'. She is concerned that the nursing profession should encourage nurses to identify their *own* nursing values, not unquestionably accept nursing values imposed from hierarchical structures. Otherwise, the full force of Thompson and Thompson's (1990) observation regarding the unconscious and early socialisation nature of our values acquisition will remain a sad unalterable truth.

In conclusion, as Steele (1986) notes, in regards to the rationale for clarifying values: 'We need a rational process so that we can take all the information we have, integrate it with our experiences, and use it knowledgeably.'

Unless we can understand and acknowledge the influences that socialisation plays in the acquisition of our values, there will be no progress in trying to *consciously* change them; for example, in the socialisation process into the nursing profession. Kelman (1966), in Yahoda and Warren's now classic work on attitudes, talks about the process of values acquisition and attitude change, where social influence encourages initial compliance with the new attitude or value; then some degree of personal identification, and only in the final instance complete internalisation of the attitude. Such a process takes varying amounts of time, and for some individuals total internalisation of values or attitudes never takes place.

There is yet another aspect to the discussion on the nature of values, namely, that for all definitions of value there is the additional characteristic of hierarchical organisation. That is, we possess several, albeit limited, values, and these we organise hierarchically, often consciously, but probably, more commonly, unconsciously.

As Omery (1989) notes, 'once a value has been integrated into this hierarchy, it has motivational worth'. Most writers on value systems agree with this statement, thus Rokeach (1973) notes 'A value system is an enduring organisation of beliefs concerning preferable modes of conduct, or end-states of existence, along a continuum of relative importance.' Silver (1976) adds 'A person's value system represents a learned organisation of values for making choices and for resolving conflicts between values!'

It would appear then, that although we may prize a particular value, it is actually present in a hierarchical system of several values, and therefore it is possible for there to be occasions when the values which we prize seem to be in conflict with each other. Thus as Omery (1989) observes, 'Intrapersonal conflict occurs when two values conflict internally for any one individual.' However, as she adds, 'While the repository of values is indeed the individual, the source of the values is usually external to the individual . . . Values are thought to be acquired through explanation, moralising, modelling, reward or punishment, identification with a person or group, or manipulation. Once acquired, they can be supported or reinforced by one's societal, peer or professional groups.' This actually can be a positive word of advice, since the better we can identify our values and thereby re-negotiate their hierarchical standing in a value-system, the better we can mobilise help, to support those values worth preserving, and encourage the development of flagging values that seem crucial to the profession (Davis, 1988).

Intrapersonal conflict of values should diminish as we re-establish the priorities of our value system, for rarely would there be simultaneously two or three competing first-class values! Omery (1989) notes, 'Professional moral values may be internalised via education or socialisation . . . whether these values become incorporated by the individual is usually a function of how closely they reflect or are an extension of earlier internalised moral values . . . A beneficial option for both the nurse and the profession is the nurse's *active and assertive involvement in the reassessment of the profession's values*' (emphasis mine).

Even if we took the example of the relative values inherent in beneficence, justice and respect for individuals so often promoted in nursing, we will find that as Abrams (1982) states 'Given the pluralistic nature of society, it is not reasonable to assume that everyone places the same value on potential harms, and benefits, and probabilities. It is therefore necessary for the physician (and the nurse) to be aware of the patient's (and their own) value system. Ignorance along these lines could be equally harmful as ignorance of medical science.' The key phrase here is *pluralistic society* and indeed many a highly valued act of beneficence has been subsequently condemned and labelled paternalistic or even outright harmful, by others. Likewise, because of our varied value-systems, what is the pursuit of justice for one individual, is often seen as gross negligence and injustice by another.

It then needs to be demonstrated that, 'One who acts unjustly from deliberation is a person who possesses in the full sense the vice of injustice, and is fully an unjust person' (Williams, 1981). This, however, is extremely rare. Usually, it is a conflict among perceived malappropriation of values that is at the root of the problem, for as Williams concludes

It is both necessary and sufficient to being a just person that one *dispositionally* promotes some courses as being just, and resists others as being unjust . . . It is not untypical of the virtues that the virtuous person should be partly characterised by the way in which he thinks about situations, and by the concepts he uses [emphasis mine].

(Williams, 1981)

We would like to think that some nursing values are shared; that there is a level at which we as nurses all agree, that some notions and occurrences are of equal value to us. This, however, is sadly not the case. There probably are very few *shared* nursing values, in spite of all our professional efforts, and certainly almost no shared international, that is, transcultural nursing values; and yet as Lanara (1988) notes 'Cultural values always have been, still are and probably will be continuously influencing the delivery of care both from the part of health care providers and the health care recipients.' Indeed, transcultural nurse theorists such as Leininger have dedicated a life's work to try and define caring modes shared by various cultures (Leininger, 1978).

Values then vary from individual to individual, but some values have more social weighting, for their manifestations in public behaviour have obvious social consequences (Steele, 1986; Ives, 1991). Kopelman (1984) in reference to the way our language, especially labelling, reflects our value system, observes that in respect of the mentally and multiply handicapped individuals, 'the language, definitions, and measures we use are shaped by our attitudes, values and interests'. She even demonstrates that 'Decisions that people are handicapped, are not value free . . . labelling others as handicapped no matter what the kind or degree, uses and creates values or obligations. If this is correct then there is no value-neutral way to describe people as handicapped and no escape from the moral responsibility of justifying these values or purposes of the ascription.' We are responsible then for the consequences of our own value-system, and this may differ sharply from the value-system of other members of society! (Farrell, 1987).

The majority of nurses work within an institution or health care structure where the values of the institution 'reflect the aggregated values of many different individuals, solidified over a significant investment of time and energy' (Omery, 1989).

It is essential to remember that even an institution's so-called values, itself represents an entire system of interlocking and inter-related values which are somewhat fuzzy at the edges, for as Inglesby (1992) comments they are 'blurred because the values and mores of society alter in patchy and straggling fashion. Values themselves, however, are only representations of larger systems of ideas which may be called philosophies or ideologies.'

When value systems conflict between an individual and the collective or the institution or profession, then inter-personal moral distress may develop. As Ives (1991) comments 'If a business or institution accepts people who hold values in conflict with those of the organisation, its ability to elicit the required individual behaviour will be weak and organisational performance will suffer.' It would not be possible, and would be of questionable utility, to only hire those individuals who agree with the institution's policies, and overriding ideology. However, knowing what the institution's values are must be helpful to some extent, thus 'to manage change, an organisation must have a well defined values statement and a mission which is understood by everyone. Awareness of an organisation's values and the assumptions the organisation makes about the external and internal environment are elements of an overall strategic plan' (Ives, 1991). Institutions need to be clear about their corporate values, and individual nurses need to be familiar with these, and their own value system, from nurse executives to the newly qualified staff nurse. As Fry (1986) comments, moral decisions in nursing are based on 'each nurse's value system – a value system in which important personal, professional and institutional values are arranged within a hierarchy of relative importance to the decision-maker.'

Deremo (1989) in an article looking at integrating professional values, quality of practice, and reimbursement, comments that 'the structure of professional nursing values, delivery of service and reimbursement systems must be addressed in order to create an institutional environment that facilitates professional nursing behaviour.'

Kramer (1974) in her now classic work on the perceptions of newly qualified staff nurses, and how they cope with the clash of values which they encounter, identifies at least three possible coping strategies; namely outward compliance, acting on principles in spite of ostracism, or a compromise situation where there is low compliance in some crucial areas and high compliance in other non-essential areas.

The whole area of conflict of values has interested poets, philosophers and ethicists for hundreds of years, as evidenced by the content of Greek dramas, where the more apparently obvious a claim of conflict of values can be raised, the greater the tragedy. Greek tragedies were rarely 'resolved' as such; all agents involved were tarnished and had to perish. Resolution came invariably from the outside. A true tragedy, a true conflict of values, according to Greek literature can never, per definition, be satisfactorily resolved.

Bernard Williams (1981), in a short essay on 'Conflict of Values' makes the essential comment and distinction between one-person value conflict and two-party value conflicts. In a truly legendary tragedy, the conflict of values is essentially intra-personal; that is, a one person conflict, although this does not hinder inter-personal values conflict from occurring simultaneously.

Philosophers have sometimes claimed that

> one-person conflict must be capable of being rationally resolved. At the very least, the theory of rational behaviour must make it an undisputed aim of the rational agent to reduce conflict in his personal set of values to the minimum. This assumption is characteristically made even by those who do not think that interpersonal conflicts of value necessarily admit of rational resolution.
>
> (Williams, 1981)

Williams (1981) points out, however, that such assumptions are themselves unreasonable. 'A characteristic dispute about values in society, such as some issue of equality against freedom, is not one most typically enacted by a body of single-minded egalitarians confronting a body of equally single-minded libertarians; but is rather a conflict which one person, equipped with a more generous range of human values, could find enacted in himself.'

More often than not, one-person value conflicts are, so-called conflicts of obligations, yet very often these, upon reflection, are only apparent *equally* binding obligations. It is not uncommon that, upon thought, one obligation takes on a more secondary position in our hierarchy of values.

It is only in the drastic, so-called tragic kind of dilemma that 'an agent can justifiably think that whatever he does will be wrong: that there are conflicting moral requirements, and that neither of them succeeds in overriding or outweighing the other'. (Williams, 1981). Some moral philosophers consider such a position as a logical inconsistency, for, they argue, how can the rational being *have* such equally pressing value claims. Surely, the rational person cannot be at war with themselves? As Williams notes (1981) 'There is a substantial and interesting question: What would have to be true of the world and of an agent that it should be impossible for him to be in a situation where whatever he did was wrong?' He actually doubts such a situation *can* naturally arise, and affirms the belief that there are apparently instances when 'there is nothing that one decently, honourably, or adequately *can* do seems a kind of truth as firmly independent of the will and inclination as anything in morality'.

According to many ethicists, values are not only plural but also in a real sense incommensurable; whereas others argue that 'unless some comparison can be made, then nothing rational can be said at all about what overall outcome is to be preferred, but more about which side of a conflict is to be chosen – and that is certainly a despairing conclusion (Williams, 1981).

Nurses profess to cherish many values, some of them chaotically placed in the hierarchy of values estimation, many of them conflicting, and several of them no longer as important as once was assumed. For some practitioners the real task ahead lies in trying to sort out the relative weightings of the values, and to reconsider why they cherish that particular set of values. For some practitioners, sorting through personal and professional values is akin to sifting through nightmares and nonsense.

Nightmares and Nonsense

Among the many attributes that can be used to describe nurses, wearing a distinctive uniform appears to be one of the most popular and enduring. Nurses wear uniforms, as doctors parade with stethoscopes around their necks, and district nurses go about the community with navy blue hats on their heads!

Such sweeping statements seem obviously inaccurate and trivial, if for no other reason than the fact that it simply is not always the case. Nonetheless, of all the recurrent topics mentioned in the nursing press, the question of uniforms, their relative benefits, use, fashion, practicality and attractiveness, is a perennial favourite (see Chapter 1).

If I were an editor of a nursing journal short on items of news, I would reach out to my five-star letterbox and pull out yet another example of nursing erudition, cap strings included! 'Sister Plume', in publishing her collected responses to letters to the editor, puts the issue of uniforms squarely under the section entitled: Perennial Preoccupations (Plume, 1988), and certainly a quick perusal of letters to the editor of our major nursing journals justifies this categorisation.

The question that needs to be addressed is not whether uniforms, as such, are of benefit to nursing, but why it is that of all the many values taken on board by the profession the question of uniforms is so deeply entrenched in complex socio-cultural, religious, historical and aesthetic justifications.

A search for a historical rationale for wearing uniforms led this writer to the early 'history' of modern nursing, military uniformity and a woman attributed with the founding of military attire, if not nursing aprons, namely 'Fiona MacNightshade' (Sellar and Yeatman, 1930). Thus we discover in Sellar and Yeatman's satire that the

> troops in the Crimea suffered terribly from cardigans and balaclava helmets and from a new kind of overcoat invented by Lord Raglan, the Commander-in-Chief. They were also only allowed to wear boots on their left feet until the memorable intervention of 'Flora MacNightlight' (the Lady with the Deadly Lampshade) who gave them boots for their right feet and other comforts and cured them of their sufferings every night with doses of deadly lampshade.
>
> (Sellar and Yeatman, 1930. Ch. 53)

Sellar and Yeatman proclaim in the introduction to their memorable book that 'Histories have previously been written with the object of exalting their authors. The object of this history is to console the reader. *No other history does this*'. Certainly Flora MacNighlight alias Flora MacNightshade, also known as Florence Nightingale, by insisting that her nurses wore a clean distinctive uniform, much akin to the prevalent attire of parlour maids of that time, ensured enduring consolation to legions of nurses ever since. (see Chapter 1). In case there is any doubt about the authenticity of Sellar and Yeatman's research, their cautionary statement in the monograph's 'Compulsory Preface' should dispel any lingering concerns, namely: 'History is not what you thought. It is what you can remember. All other history defeats itself,' (Sellar and Yeatman, 1930).

In the domain of values, it is not what is really the case that is of primary importance. Rather, what counts as important is what we endow with value. Thus, nurses attribute importance to uniforms because they want uniforms to be of value and importance to them.

'Sister Plume' eloquently speaks for generations of nurses when she states that 'one of the greatest satisfactions for me was donning uniform for the first time. In those days when we put on our uniforms we *felt* somebody, and no grenadier guardsman – nor the Lord Mayor himself – could feel a greater pride than that which rose in our bosoms.' (Plume, 1988).

She then proceeds to disclose the central secret embedded in the 'uniform controversy', namely: 'What cared we that our lot was the humble proba-tioner's single stripe? For the world and his wife we were *nurses*, and we had taken our first step on the road that would lead us to the coveted lace cap of the staff nurse, and we could perhaps dream of the day we might don the sacred navy blue of the Sister' (Plume, 1988).

Uniforms have value to nurses and are precious status symbols because they represent authority and power, if not a form of distinctness. It is considered important to separate nurses from patients – 'and if you have any doubts about the truth of this, you have only to walk on those misguided psychiatric wards where uniform has been dispensed with: what with patients wearing their outdoor clothes, and nurses in mufti, it is almost impossible to tell patients and nursing staff apart! And then where are you?' (Plume, 1988).

It is interesting to note that it was precisely psychiatric nurses who not without great effort and amid much controversy, first abandoned the wearing of a distinctive uniform, and this in spite of some notable sociological research which demonstrated that once a person is inside a psychiatric hospital (with a psychiatric diagnosis) it is almost impossible to shift that diagnosis, even in the presence of perfectly 'normal' behaviour and absence of mental or organic disease! (Rosenhan, 1973) It is very easy to be confused as to relative role status in a psychiatric unit, but the plunge having been taken, the psychiatric community has never looked back. It is not the uniform that is therapeutic, but the person who wears it.

'Sister Plume' contends that there is value in 'singling out special groups of individuals by some tangible code of dress and we would do well to recognise the importance of this essentially human tradition, especially as . . . uniform has such an utilitarian purpose' (Plume, 1988).

Finding utilitarian purposes in a nurse's uniform is a bit like justifying the purchase of a new car. There may be many good and valid reasons why we choose to buy a new car but ultimately we do so for one overriding reason – because we choose to do so. Thus, we could say, nurses continue to wear uniforms, some of which are most impractical, because they choose to do so, or because nursing managers wish that their employees continue to wear them. In fact 'Sister Plume' may well be correct in stating that 'one of the most important elements in the uniform is preventing staff from looking the same' (Plume, 1988), and nurse managers often find the adoption of distinctive uniforms by various members of staff a quick guide to 'skills mix and competency'. It is reassuring no doubt to the busy, harassed sister that she has four nurses on duty, namely – two stripes, a belt and a string! Unfortunately as 'Sister Plume' observed, apart from some specialist hospitals, 'the grace of the London hospital's special headgear has followed the starch apron into obscurity and we are all the poorer for it'. 'Sister Plume' challenges nursing leaders to explain why they banished the cap and the apron, 'where was the referendum on the starched apron and how came you to withdraw it from service without the agreement of the practising nurse?'

Even student nurses consider the distinctive nurses uniform as being functional and full of professional value, that is *valuable*; thus, 'we should not be afraid of maintaining our professional identity by wearing a distinctive uniform. Far from blocking communication with patients, the uniform is of therapeutic advantage. It gives great reassurance to patients' (Lockley, 1992). This is an interesting statement, no doubt from a devotee of 'Sister Plume'. Patients may well need reassurance as to a nurse's competency and abilities, but by far the overwhelming mass of evidence attests to the fact that it is not necessarily a uniform that instills this confidence and reassurance in a frightened patient. There are on the contrary instances when a distinctive, traditional uniform is patently inadvisable, for example in paediatrics or some of the specialty areas, such as oncology nursing, intensive care, theatre nursing or community nursing.

Nurses that claim uniforms to have quasi-magical powers of healing and therapeutic intervention are usually looking at a very narrow definition of nursing practice, and are desperately trying to justify why they hold the nurse's uniform of paramount value. Such justifications sound very similar to the loud protestations of a six year old, that '*all* the kids on the street have roller skates'. Such statements as '*many* nurses believe we should abandon the awful national uniform and return to hats and traditional uniforms . . . please let us learn to be *real* nurses, and to wear a uniform that allows us to look like real nurses' (Lockley, 1992, emphasis mine) call for closer scrutiny. With great horror the student nurse observes that 'some hospitals have abandoned the use of hats, and there have been suggestions that nurses on general wards should not wear uniforms as they are thought to be a barrier to communication' (Lockley, 1992).

Whether or not uniforms are a barrier to communication needs to be determined by research and by observing nurses communicating on the wards with patients, staff, relatives and students. Observing nurses 'communicating' on a ward is a little like observing water babies at play, where, 'to prove no water babies exist, one must see no water babies existing, which is not the same thing as not seeing water babies' (Kingsley, 1986). Much anecdotal evidence exists that either supports the wearing of uniforms or advocates its abolition. All the literature supports the claim that of prime importance in the debate is nurses' *feelings and attitudes* toward the uniform, which is a question of personal preference and value rather than irrefutable research evidence that wearing or discarding a uniform is a professional benefit or loss. Thus, a registered nurse, in a letter to the editor of a nursing journal states 'Many nurses now *feel* that this was a great mistake and that we should again wear caps . . . we *feel* that a return to wearing caps would enhance and complete our professional appearance and would therefore encourage hospitals to retain caps for their nurses' (Wright, 1992).

Nurse Wright is concerned with her professional appearance, while the Elderly Care Co-ordinator for Darlington Health Authority is concerned with promoting patient-staff interaction. 'Far from making it difficult for residents and relatives to identify nurses, wearing mufti will allow nurses to project their own personality and develop closer relationships with patients' (Browne, 1992). Likewise, Glasper and Miller (1992) suggest that paediatric nurses leave their uniforms at home, and adopt colourful, practical work clothing, which should increase work satisfaction, access to patients and patient/family co-operation with nursing care. As the two researchers note, 'The change in uniform has created a more relaxed atmosphere in the children's unit. Although there is *no empirical evidence*, staff working in the new-look uniforms report an overall improvement in communication with families and other professional groups' (emphasis mine).

It will be interesting to follow up paediatric nurses who move from traditional uniforms to colourful practical work clothes, and the difference this makes to patient care. Certainly in modern paediatrics the common trait among child health nurses of putting the child and its family at the centre of one's concern has led to the supreme value of openness and adaptability 'a willingness to adopt new innovations which can be shown to be of benefit to the client group' (Glasper and Miller, 1992).

It is not clear, however, why in some nursing groups creativity and a penchant for taking risks (if there is reasonable evidence of the benefits to patients outweighing any other value or consideration) are more noticeable than in others. Where the wearing of uniforms is concerned, the doubt justly creeps in that more is being discussed than simply clothing, as 'Sister Plume' exclaims 'I am proud of my uniform and it is a pride redoubled whenever a bus conductor says "Good morning, Sister", or I am recognised by a former patient in the grocers' (Plume, 1988).

One wonders what 'Sister Plume' would have to say about the Southampton experiment or Sparrow's (1991) work with general nurses, since her advice is 'to wear your uniform with pride and, above all, to resist all temptations to venture into trousers' (Plume, 1988).

The nurse's uniform, as any uniform, is as much a symbol of the work performed by the wearer as a proof of status and entitlement to privileges. The 'impedimenta' as Glasper and Miller refer to watch and pencils, etc. can be as well carried in the universal American style 'bum-bag' as they do on the paediatric wards in Southampton, as wear them pinned onto the uniform (Glasper and Miller, 1992). Plume claims, as do many nurses, that wearing these attributes of power and practice looks impressive – 'State Registration badge, School of Nursing badge, fob watch, scissors chain, pan clip, pan torch, spatula and Spencer-Wells forceps, no wonder we enjoyed universal respect when we projected such a readiness for any eventuality' (Plume, 1988).

The real hidden agenda, however, behind insisting that nurses wear a particular uniform is that the wearer of the uniform can hide her inadequacies behind the facade of uniform clothing, specific to rank and function; as 'Plume' would say, 'What is good enough for the Duke of Wellington is good enough for the foot soldier' (Plume, 1988). Indeed uniforms in the nursing profession were introduced, military style, in the context of strict hierarchical practice and blind obedience to superiors (Jolley, 1989). Individuality was consciously discouraged and it was certainly not the intention to ease practice or facilitate patient communication, probably American ideas anyway; 'one never has to look very far for an American influence in the more lunatic reaches of the world of nursing' (Plume, 1988).

Nurse Education, Project 2000, Post Registration Education

The effects of change in nursing could be mirrored in this conversation piece familiar to many from childhood literature:

> 'Who are *you*?' said the caterpillar. Alice replied, rather shyly, 'I – hardly know sir, just at present – at least I knew who I *was* when I got up this morning, but I think I must have been changed several times since then.' 'What do you mean by that?' said the caterpillar sternly. 'Explain yourself'. 'I can't explain *myself* I'm afraid, sir', said Alice, 'because I'm not myself you see.' 'I don't see', said the caterpillar.
>
> (Carroll, 1968; ch. V)

That nurse education has gone through, and is currently undergoing, major changes, is an enormous understatement. That nurses needed a new emphasis in their preparation and education for professional nursing in the twenty-first century is also self-evident. What is less clear is the rationale for the intensity of emotions that discussion of nurse preparation engenders, the nature of values surrounding the issue of nurse preparation, continuing education of practising nurses, and the values manifest when second level nurses convert to registration status. What are the values inherent in nurse education? To what extent do we transmit them consciously and overtly, and to what extent are they part of an elaborate socialisation process conveyed potently and covertly?

In an interesting report on changing values of new nursing students over a period of ten years, Garvin and Boyle (1985) found that the high economic value orientation they identified was consistent with other studies that showed greater concern, now, with work security and economic stability than in previous years. This shift in concern comes after social, religious and aesthetic values; a triad of values unchanged from a similar study a decade previously. Interestingly, economic concerns have taken precedence over political and theoretical values in nursing. As the researchers note, if these are the basic entering values of prospective nursing students (albeit in this example, American students) these findings 'have implications for student selection and retention, curriculum design and the establishment of a learning environment which reinforces and highlights values associated with a humanistic and scientific discipline'.

Nurse preparation is designed for the most part by non-practising theoretical, educationalist nurses, however, and therefore, not only are the values of entering students (probably values resembling most closely what the public thinks about nursing) not taken into account, but not developed any further either. The new values imposed and instilled into nursing students are as frightening and as far reaching in their effects as any values imposed on previous generations by 'Sister Plume' and her cohorts. As Garvin and Boyle (1985) note: 'Nursing needs to deliberately select and retain a rich variety of students and to produce graduates that reflect these values.' However, this must be done without brutalising nursing students in the process.

The nursing profession has values it wishes to transmit to its members and which it desires its members to uphold, therefore, not surprisingly Garvin and Boyle (1985) note 'Nurse educators need to monitor the characteristics of entering students to effectively influence the qualities congruent with contemporary nursing.' The question remains, however, what do we do with 'non-congruent values' and who decides which values are 'nursing' values and which are not? The two researchers add: 'Students need assistance clarifying their values and appropriate career guidance . . . the practice setting must reinforce these values.' However, it would sometimes appear as if it were not at all obvious what values were being installed, inculturated, perpetuated or even eradicated. The advice of the Duchess to Alice in Wonderland could well apply to many a nursing novice:

'Be what you would seem to be', or if you'd like it put more simply, 'Never imagine yourself not to be otherwise than what it might appear to others that what you were or might have been was not otherwise than what you had been would have appeared to them to be otherwise.'

(Carroll, 1968; ch. IX)

The first task therefore facing the nurse educationalist is to decide where he/she wishes nursing to go. Some decisions have already been made, based on societal needs and growing pressures for change within the profession itself if it is to respond adequately to modern demands. It is important, however, that not only nurse educationalists, nurse managers, nurse theorists and nurse practitioners but also students of nursing and the general public, understands and knows where the nursing profession is heading. Otherwise, we may well be re-enacting the classic scene of Alice in Wonderland when she asks the Cheshire Cat for directions:

'Would you please tell me, please, which way I ought to go from here?'
'That depends a good deal on where you want to get to', said the Cat.
'I don't much care where – ' said Alice.
'Then it doesn't matter which way you go', said the Cat.
' – so long as I get somewhere', Alice added as an explanation.
'Oh, you're sure to do that', said the Cat, 'if you only walk long enough.'

(Carroll, 1968; ch VI)

Alice does not know where she is going, all she wants to do is to 'get somewhere', a compulsion to move and change at any cost. This insistent movement and change in the health care field is a frequent phenomenon, change for the sake of change, possibly to satisfy the goals and needs of administrators and managers, but extremely stressful and wasteful of resources for practitioners, educators and nursing students (see Chapter 5).

Modern nursing wishes to be more academically sound, for it claims that an increased knowledge base will put nursing practice in a better position to be intelligently implemented. This more in-depth knowledge of man's health, environment, nursing theory and understanding of man's bio-psycho-social and spiritual being, is to take place in an atmosphere of freedom, choice and learning. Raya (1990), in an interesting article challenging nurse educators to consider whether nursing knowledge can be promoted while nursing values are ignored, reminds the reader that the advanced new nurse education that is currently taking place in colleges of higher education, polytechnics and universities will now be joining the rest of academia in sharing in the fruits of its lengthy experience.

Raya sees the university as 'the cradle which nurtures the intellectuals, professionals, researchers, leaders, state servants, academic scientists and others. It promotes the whole cycle of sciences and is a source of spiritual and cultural radiation.' This is a very positive image of the role and function of a university, one which she adds has the 'formative power, shaping personalities and cultivating the desire of perfection' (Raya, 1990). This, however, may be seen by many a nurse educator and senior nursing practitioner as usurping *their* hitherto firmly held function and prerogative. Raya points out that the 'purpose of the university is to cultivate the attitudes and the traits of character which symbolise the educated mind'. What nursing needs to determine is which traits of character it wishes its students and practitioners to cultivate.

The author of this chapter still remembers words addressed to her not quite a decade ago that, after all, she need not be concerned with *that*, for she was not there to think! Such a comment begs comparison with Alice's experiences at the court of the Red and White Queen where she observes: "'I've a right to think", said Alice sharply, for she was beginning to feel a little worried. "Just about as much right", said the Duchess, "as pigs have to fly."' (Carroll, 1968; ch. IX)

Not only does nursing need to be consistent in the messages it is aiming to transmit, but also clear about the limits it is not prepared to transgress. Universities and academic institutions attempt to provide an atmosphere where students can grow and develop intellectually, often along the path of trial and error, mistakes and blind alleys. Nursing, however, holding perfection as a high value is reluctant to forego previous practices and is the antithesis of risk taking. It avoids confrontations, (especially of practice) and is merciless towards any evidence of imperfection or mistake. Hinkle et al. (1982) asked mathematics-anxious adults about to undertake a course of behavioural statistics 'How do you feel when you make mistakes?' for he found that his own reply to the question was not shared by his students, namely that: 'I find my mistakes interesting and my confusions even more so . . . mistakes are like windows into our minds' (Hinkle et al. 1982). This is a splendid attitude toward learning in the Greek sense of academia that Raya (1990) was referring to, but a far cry from the practice reality of nursing; where giving a patient an extra vitamin tablet is after penalised in the same way as giving an overdose of insulin. Fortunately, practice *is* slowly changing, but with increased responsibility, and without an increase in knowledge base, many nurses are finding that they are indeed making grave mistakes, and these mistakes are pursued relentlessly. As the mathematics teacher would accede, it all depends on the nature of the mistake. Some mistakes are unforgivable, because they violate *more* than the fashionable rule which prizes knowledge above all else. Such a deficiency can be easily rectified, as is evidenced by a plethora of continuing nursing education courses, but if the mistake demonstrates an absence of primary nursing value such as a caring attitude, compassion, or patience, the resulting puishment can be devastating and remorseless.

When nurses transgress the norms of behaviour and face the wrath of their seniors and professional leaders, they are understandably devastated. Help must be made available for these nurses if we are to really enact the values of consideration and concern which we profess to possess. As Baly (1984; p. 10) points out, 'It is important that not only is help available but that it is known to be available. Nurses have attempted suicide in despair, not because the help they needed was not there, but because they did not know it was there.'

We are nonetheless, as a profession, unforgiving of mistakes, possibly understandably; as Baly (1984; p. 5) notes 'If professionals have an implied contract with society which gives them "status, authority and privilege" then society wants certain assurances in return.'

What do we do with those who transgress our norms over major nursing values? In the recent incident over the case of a paediatric nurse manager who was caught indecently assaulting young children, the legal establishment found him guilty and prosecuted him accordingly. The UKCC Professional Conduct

Committee, however, found him guilty of misconduct, but did *not* revoke his registration, sparking off a debate that is still raging among general nurses, paediatric nurses and the public at large. An interesting article (Long, 1992) trying to analyse the rationale behind the UKCC decision has only served to rekindle the debate answering few of the questions posed, and possibly violating the right to privacy of the offending nurse. True, some wrongs are so great, the profession must disassociate itself from the perpetrators of such deeds, but does this imply that the nurse in question should therefore have to face ridicule, derision and professional ostracism (having served his prison sentence) for the rest of his life? There is no model answer to such terrible questions; one thing is sure, however, the issues raised speak to the core and essence of nursing. Nursing values are being scrutinised, examined, and in some instances found wanting.

Thoreau (1960) commenting on the functioning of governments notes: 'Government is at best an expedient, but most governments are usually, and all governments are sometimes, inexpedient.' I fear that the same could be said of nursing leadership and some of the values they appear to espouse. The solution of course is for nurses to take a more active role in supporting and helping to shape the thinking of its leadership. Thoreau (1960) continues 'Let every man make known what kind of government would command his respect, and that will be one step forward to obtaining it' for 'a corporation has no conscience, but a corporation of conscientious men is a corporation with a conscience' (Thoreau, 1960) (see also Chapter 5).

A review of nursing final examination papers over the years illustrates well the changing values in nursing as reflected in nurse education. In 1925 the General Nursing Council for England and Wales (GNC) Final State Examinations for the General Register, asked the students to define Chorea, describing the symptoms and usual treatment; to enumerate the varieties of fractures, 'giving a short description of each' and to describe the cause of uterine haemorrhage. All this in the space of 90 minutes! It brings to mind other impossible endeavours expected of the naive student such as Sellar and Yeatman's (1930) spoof question 6b from Test paper V 'Up to End of History: Did anybody say "I know that no-one can save this country and that nobody else can?" If not, who did say it?' Such impossible tasks are still asked of students but at least in the context of nursing studies they are more likely to be asked about *nursing* undertakings, not medical diagnosis.

In 1929 questions asked under the heading of Surgery and Surgical Nursing referred to an aural discharge in a 6 year old and the likely advice to the mother (one dreads to think what the nurse was expected to do), while a question on when a bladder washout may be prescribed is in the section on gynaecology nursing! Nonetheless, advice to a distraught mother and performing a bladder washout are both accepted practices in *nursing* even today. No sooner had the student nurse answered these questions than she was then given a second paper, also of 90 minutes duration, on medicine and medical nursing. Question two asked in what conditions were the following drugs commonly ordered, Atropine, Camphore, Jalap, Ergot and Laudanum, making amusing reading today, but how many of our current graduates could describe the pharmokinetics of commonly used drugs today?

The next question asked about Insulin, which in a paper set in 1928 was very progressive and commendable. How many nurses today could describe the indications, side-effects and nursing implications for practice of Cyclosporin, Acyclovir or even AZT, all more common today than Insulin was in 1928!

Increasingly, the questions asked for *nursing* knowledge and *nursing implications* of medical protocols, even if this was not made explicit. Some questions still had a Sellar and Yeatman feel to them, for example, 'Mention all the conditions you know for which it may be desirable to feed a patient entirely by the rectum' or 'At what temperature should the following be prepared: cold, tepid and hot baths?' Some questions a contemporary oncology post-registration student would find difficulty in answering, such as 'What are the chief differences between simple and malignant tumours? or How does a malignant tumour destroy life?' The really fascinating point to ponder is not the overtly medical nature of the questions but that they were asked in the first place.

In 1933, Oncology as a medical science was in its infancy and nursing boards were asking questions the equivalent of aspects of gene therapy or *in vitro* fertilisation today. Perhaps these questions were rarely attempted and poorly answered, but the educational message was that nurses must be proficient for current and forward-looking practice. How many student nurses today read scientific journals, even the more popular ones such as *New Scientist*, *Scientific American* or the science/medical sections of the serious press? Universities and higher education institutions should be encouraging students to seek out such information and endeavour to teach them how and where to locate the answers to the many questions that practice may suggest. In this task adequate libraries are essential in promoting this value.

By 1938 questions were distinctly more community orientated; for example, on vaccination, advice to parents for a child discharged home following the setting of a fractured arm, description of enuresis, and ingrowing toenails. Also posed were some purely nursing questions such as 'How would you proceed to tepid sponge a patient for the reduction of temperature?'

The war years brought, not surprisingly, questions about thrombosis, delirium and blood transfusions. By 1952 progress in science and technology was reflected in questions on antibiotic drug treatments and conditions requiring catheterisation. Male nurses were still set separate papers (on venereal and genito-urinary diseases), but the papers were now being set by a joint board of medical and *nursing* representatives.

Factors that predispose to pressure sores and their prevention was one of the topics in 1954, and in 1966 to list the possible causes of mental confusion in the elderly after admission to hospital, and to give details of the nursing management of such patients. Without adequate access to nursing research which was then in its embryonic stages, it is interesting to ponder on the nature of these questions and their possible answers.

Creeping into the examinations are concerns for nurses' safety; for example, aspects of avoiding 'back strain' and prevention of iatrogenic infections. Social concerns are evident also, such as maternity provisions for pregnant women (although this was a question posed on the 1962 *experimental* syllabus paper).

In the 1970s nursing students were asked about oral hygiene and evidence of an understanding on the role and function of *other* members of the health care team. Just fourteen years ago, nurses sitting the final paper for Registered Mental Handicap Nursing sat a paper, set entirely by expert nurses in the field, and were asked to comment on moves to relocate patients from large institutions to housing in the community.

Psychiatric nurses in the early eighties were expected to understand aspects of care for a mentally disturbed sexual offender, effects of institutionalisation on patients, the nature of the grieving process, hyperaction, and the role of the community psychiatric nurse in relation to promotion of mental health.

Clearly, as nursing education concerns reflect a change from a medical model to a nursing paradigm so the nursing questions posed in final examinations reflected increasingly societal concerns, scientific innovations, community responsiveness and limits of professional responsibility.

Currently, however, nursing education is being torn asunder by a seemingly incompatible set of values. Nursing educational leaders would like to promote androgogical approaches to nurse education (not without protests from some student quarters). As one nursing student noted: 'An adult response from a tutor depends upon adult input from a student' (Allen, 1992). At the same time widening the entry gate for nurse education is potentially a recipe for disaster. On the one hand, nurse educationalists aspire to instil into neophyte nurses humanistic values and an appreciation of the fine arts, especially as they impinge on the art of nursing; on the other hand, time, money and lack of intellectual resources among the educators themselves means that the students are being offered disjointed programmes, consisting of the intellectual highlights (or in some instances titbits) of the social and humanistic sciences. The curricula are 'busy' and phrenetic and no time is made available for the student to 'stand and stare'. As Thoreau observed two hundred years ago 'Most men, even in this comparatively free country, through more ignorance and mistake are so occupied with the factitious cares and superfluously coarse labours of life that its fine fruits cannot be plucked by them.' (Thoreau, 1960).

Academia should be about taking time out to think and reflect, yet pre-registration programmes although aiming and aspiring to this goal consist largely of highly planned activities geared toward helping novice nurses understand and adapt to the *practice* of nursing. The nurse of the twenty-first century is only going to be a 'knowledgeable doer' to the extent that 'knowing' influences her 'doing'. The question yet to be answered is what does the nurse of the twenty-first century need to know, what are her sources of knowing, and what does she do with her knowledge? Again, it is Thoreau, the archetypal homespun philosopher who notes: 'How can he remember well his ignorance – which his growth requires – who has so often to use his knowledge?' (Thoreau, 1960).

In the process of maturing professionally we forget our blunders, mistakes and inaccuracies, even though we had to go through them, acknowledge and accept them in order to proceed further. Today's virtues are built on the vices of yesterday, and often it is our awareness of the maturation process and all that it entails, that tempts us to reject the conforming outcome. Thus as Thoreau wryly comments, 'The greater part of what my neighbours call good I believe in my soul to be bad, and if I repent of anything, it is very likely to be my good behaviour. What demon possessed me that I behaved so well?' (Thoreau, 1960).

In a study looking at professional values of English nursing undergraduates, two themes were identified as being of most significance, namely (a) respect of persons and (b) being able to take time over 'little things' (Kelly, 1991). English nursing students were concerned that humanistic orientations permeate not only their gestalt but also their professional lives, respecting patients was about 'the way you actually treat patients'.

It is interesting that one of the most powerful mechanisms to manifest this care and respect towards a patients was seen to be the possibly enviable luxury of having time to think about little things. Students expressed this phenomenon as 'worrying about people's glasses, where their teeth are or who will feed their cat while they are in the hospital' (Kelly, 1991). They identify the expert nurses, as those nurses who are 'good role models . . . people that you have looked up to and said "That's the kind of nurse I'd like to be . . . that's how it should be done . . . spending time . . . just in little things" (Kelly, 1991). As one student observed, as you watch your expert nurse performing personal hygiene with a patient, and she is combing her hair "and they get a mirror out so that the patient can just look at themselves". It's *mostly an approach* you can pick up from some people' (Kelly, 1991) (emphasis mine).

As Kelly notes, for the students the opposite of this approach is 'cutting corners'; no deep seated malice, but simply a slovenly approach to care, fostered by low staff morale, high patient-staff ratios, increased patient morbidity and therefore dependency on the staff, and finally higher throughput of patients which discourages establishing bonds and leaving the time to 'wonder'. One articulate student put the issue very succinctly, as follows:

> The biggest problem I find is the pressure to get through the work . . . There is not much positive reinforcement . . . you don't have time to think . . . you don't think of what you are doing, you just want to finish . . . Also, nobody's going to know . . . Like, for example, an older person . . . nobody's going to know if you took the extra minute to offer them a choice of clothes because it takes so much time. You have to smile and look as if you really want them to choose. The only person that is going to make you do it is your own conscience.
>
> (Kelly, 1991)

It is sad to reflect that the above was said by a nursing student, who should be in the honeymoon period of her professional life. As one nursing student observed 'Nurses haven't got the power to change the situation they are in at the moment. It's a massive traditional thought within nursing . . . and it won't change until it has changed itself' (Kelly, 1991). Therefore the students add, you may have to modify your values, 'not that you leave your standards behind, but you have to modify them a bit', 'You pick up values . . . but you make a conscious effort to say, "Look, I am keeping my head down and I am working but I am still going to keep my own self-identity and the values that are mine"' (Kelly, 1991).

The student nurse is defiant and claiming as her own prerogative, power to think and behave as she chooses. Glen (1990), however, emphatically declares that 'there is no serious and sustained analysis of power in the literature of nursing education'. A pity since all our behaviour and motivations behind our actions are controlled by varying degrees of power relationships, as noted, to their cost by Kelly's research subjects. 'Power relations are not simply chosen by nurse teachers but made more or less necessary by the organisational structure under which they come together '(Glen, 1990). Nurse teachers, however, need to develop the students capacity 'for critical reflection and freedom from habit, precedent, coercion and self-deception'. A daunting task at the best of times. It is the hidden values and conflicting values that hinder progress most effectively.

Glen (1990) looking at reasons why schools and colleges of nursing may be thwarting the development of nursing students, cites the educationalist Stenhouse (1982), One of the central problems relating to curriculum innovation is that social and political life in colleges of nursing, as elsewhere, depends on the unspoken agreement and the 'hidden cards'. The 'unspoken agreement' among nursing educationalists and theorists appears to be a desperate attempt at modern, progressive, thought-and-act conformity, not dissimilar in its extreme position from the rigidity of the past. A serious case of 'the emperor's new clothes'. The remedy for this disease, is to only promulgate what is reasonably sound, proven or shown to be effective by intellectual analysis, research and *practice*. As Glen (1990) notes, 'what this suggests is that the path to an effective powerbase in nursing education must be trod by intellectual and practitioner together'.

The development, according to Glen, of 'climates which encourage and support individual and collective reflective practice and value and promote [the] intra professional critical thinking and questioning' needs to be addressed. Such a scenario would demand that *value* is placed on pluralism as an intrinsic quality (emphasis mine). Nursing students with values different from those of the prevailing nursing workforce should be listened to and encouraged to develop in the interest of the whole profession, if not better patient care. Glen warns nurse educationalists that 'Nursing education must perform its own institutions and create new structures and strategies more congruent with the notion of professionalism. If it cannot realise these reforms, it will never gain the power it constantly seeks.'

Allen (1992), a Project 2000 nursing student, notes that 'the mythology attached to nursing affects how we *expect* to be treated. In our fantasies we have not moved far from the era of the strident matron and the dragon ward sister and a system of training that existed to support this regime of compliance.' Glen would sympathise with this student, encouraging qualified nurses to base the source of their power on genuine expertise, openness, and a willingness to exchange ideas; the archetypal academic university climate (see also Chapter 4.)

Ironically, it is in the advent of 'academic' nursing, a pursuit of 'theory' and research-based practice that has highlighted some of the most blatant idiosyncrasies and faults of the academic system itself. As Auld (1992) observes 'We are, however, in danger of adopting every idea and buzz word that arrives from across the Atlantic in the belief that their application *must* improve patient care' [emphasis mine]. One of the most powerful forces to influence English nursing in the past twenty years is the development from Northern America of nursing theories, models and a blind insistence that everything from soaps to bedcovers, dressings to advice, be research-based and research-validated. As Auld (1992) notes, 'It is fatuous to concentrate on making nurses technically competent through a training programme if at the same time we encourage them to be intellectually inept. Education and practice must reinforce each other.' As Auld rightfully concludes, 'To prevent delays in progress in the future, we need to question why the profession has indulged in this flirtation with academia, without engagement.' I would even add, without valid engagement.

The practising non-university trained nurse tends to look askance at so called degree nurses, provoking immediate knee-jerk responses from such qualified members of the profession. Thus, 'I resent being told that my nursing care is not good enough to work in a hands-on setting. If it is not good enough for that, then it is certainly not good enough for teaching or research' (Matthew, 1992) and 'Let us remember that we are all nurses. If this is not good enough ground for mutual respect then I will start to feel ashamed of being a nurse.' (Ellis, 1992).

Practising nurses are suspicious of academically prepared nurses and reluctant to take on board research findings as such, because they have an understandable fear of the unknown in academia, especially nursing academia, which has promoted much that is of questionable value to the nursing profession. Any serious questioning of the professional utility of some novel nursing theories, models or research activities, meets however, with immediate condemnation, if not frowning and disdain. If nursing is to really enter into the academic arena, it must be prepared for dissent, discussion, debate and maverick loners. Plato has Socrates commenting that 'the things approved by the lover of wisdom and discussion are most valid and true' (*Republic*: IX: 583, In Hamilton and Cairns, 1961); but this does not mean that just because something is approved by an academician it is by this approbation endowed with additional magic-like qualities. In reference to admiration and approval, if not outright love, Socrates observes to Euthyphro, 'It is not because a thing is loved that they who love it love it, but it is loved because they love it' (*Euthyphro*: 11, In Hamilton and Cairns 1961). Likewise, learning and scholarship are admired not because it is ipso facto, admirable, but because it is worth admiring.

Scholarship, (even nursing scholarship) should be pursued, not because it is the legitimate pursuit of intelligent nurses, but because scholarship may contain, reveal or encourage truths that enlighten and shape practice. If they are not seen to do this or are not seen to be contributing to the debate concerning the nature of nursing arts and sciences, maybe we should consider abandoning those particular avenues of thought. As King observes: 'If theory is not useful it really is not worth the effort to develop it' (King, 1971;p. 16). This may take more courage than to be seen not approving blanketly all that we hear and read. Continuing his discussion with Euthyphro, Socrates, foreseeing this line of argument notes: 'Where, however, you have reverence, there you have fear as well. Is there anybody who has reverence and a sense of shame about an act, and does not at the same time dread and fear an evil reputation?' (*Euthyphro*, 12c, In Hamilton and Cairns, 1961).

It is considered enlightened to accept nursing theories, models and conceptual frameworks; so much so, that to query some of their underlying assumptions and prototypic theories is perceived as iconoclastic. Yet as Johnson (1990) observes, 'the models of nursing advanced so far deal in only very superficial ways with moral questions and, as frameworks for thought and subsequent action, they are full of contradictions, jargon and are untested in clinical reality'.

Nurses studying these issues are in awe of the content and terrified to voice an opposition or query an operative premise. The result is a situation akin to the story of the emperor and his new clothes. Who will be the child to burst the bubble? Who will be the boy David to topple Goliath? All aspects of nursing theories need to be challenged, but only some aspects have obvious immediate flaws.

One of the most persistently quoted inadequacies of the theory presentation debate is the language used to elucidate the readership. (King, 1971; p.10). In *Alice in Wonderland* the Eaglet unceremoniously announces '"Speak English!' said the Eaglet. 'I don't know the meaning of half those long words and what's more I don't believe you do either!"' (Carroll, 1968; Ch. 3).

Unfortunately, nurses rarely seem so emphatic, they prefer to vote with their feet (or minds) and simply side-step the entire issue, while enduring linguistic agonies in muted silence. In fact, talk of models of nursing causes as much visible effect on practising staff nurses as Alice's effect on the mouse by persistent mention of Dinah, her cat!

Not only is language obscure and obtuse, it tends to be inconsistent and disorganised. What one theoretician calls a model of nursing, another refers to as a theory, conceptual framework, even sometimes a paradigm or meta paradigm. To query the inconsistencies of language application is to be considered 'uninformed' or somehow academically slothful. It is the little ones of this world, however, that demonstrate the appropriateness of timeless truths, and thus we smile in agreement at the conversation between the members of the Mad Hatter's tea party:

'Then you should say what you mean', the March Hare went on.
'I do', Alice hastily replied; 'at least I mean what I say – that's the same you know.'
'Not the same thing a bit!', said the Hatter.
'Why, you might just as well say that "I see what I eat!" is the same thing as "I eat what I see!"'
'You might just as well say', added the March Hare, 'that "I like what I get" is the same thing as "I get what I like!"'

(Carroll, 1968; ch. VII).

Usage of words needs to be consistent if they are to convey any genuine meaning and thereby promote ideas, instigate debate and discussion, and challenge the status quo. Unfortunately, as Thoreau noted in 1840 to his sorrow: 'We love eloquence for its own sake, and not for any truth which it may utter, or any heroism it may inspire' (Thoreau, 1960). Many a nurse, having come to terms with the theoretical bases of the nursing process, may be tempted to repeat happily after the Red Queen, having just read a few passages from nursing theory expositions "'You may call it 'nonsense' if you like", she said, "but I've heard nonsense compared with which that would be as sensible as a dictionary!'" (Carroll, 1968; ch. 2).

Some theoreticians are concerned with the looseness with which words are applied to perceived phenomena, for example Smith (1990) drawing attention to the raging debate over the use and meaning of the word 'caring'. One wonders, however, to what extent she made her comments because she saw herself in a different intellectual camp, rather than for a genuine concern over the use of gerunds in correct English grammar or event in an attempt to continue the academic debate over the semantics involved.

Again, it is our dream characters that find the courage to say what we inwardly suspect: 'When I use a word", Humpty Dumpty said, in rather a scornful tone, "it means must what I choose it to mean – neither more nor less'" (Carroll, 1968; ch. 6). Presumably, like Humpty Dumpty, the more a word has to 'work' the higher its salary – thus 'When I make a word do a lot of work like that', said Humpty Dumpty, 'I always pay it extra'" (Carroll, 1968; ch. 6). A quick review of the cost of some of the books on nursing theories and monographs on nursing models would seem to support this absurd observation, but then in nursing matters things get 'curioser and curioser' and staying with academic nursing surely prompts the observation that one must be mad. 'How do you know I'm mad?', said Alice. 'You must be', said the Cat, 'or you wouldn't have come here' (Carroll, 1968; ch. 11).

The current effort to improve standards in nursing practice via continuing education, upgrading of enrolled nurses to registered nurse status by conversion courses, and the introduction of Project 2000 courses, and so on, all give the impression of motion, commotion and ant-like activity. The Red Queen's comments: 'here you see, it takes all the running you can do, to keep in the same place. If you want to get somewhere else, you must run at least twice as fast as that!' (Carroll, 1968; ch. 2) can surely be echoed up and down the land by many an exhausted, struggling nurse. Not that only nursing students and nurses pursuing part-time studies feel this way. Staff nurses and educators are feeling tired and stressed when asked by health care management and even society at large to perform the impossible, if not small miracles. Protestations that what is asked for is impossible, that such cutting of corners and dilution of practice by increasing volume is unprofessional, tend to go unheeded. Rather practitioners are told by their managers to attend in addition to their usual work, assertiveness courses, time management courses, fill out forms to demonstrate the level of their busyness and to input information onto computers so that it can be demonstrated that the practitioner is indeed adequately occupied! To this Alice (the nurses) protestations go unheeded. "'There's no use trying", she said, "one can't believe impossible things." "I daresay you haven't had much practice", said the Queen. "When I was your age I always did it for half an hour a day. Why, sometimes I've believed as many as six impossible things before breakfast'" (Carroll, 1968; ch. 5).

Current NHS reforms and nursing education policies ask the profession not only to believe in six impossible things before breakfast, but to implement them by tea-time. No longer has the profession the luxury of time and discussion, bearing in mind Alice's observation that even when one does voice queries and concerns, they may go unlistened to, but how can you talk with a person if they always say the same thing?' (Carroll, 1968; ch. 5).

Thoreau (1960) speaks so eloquently for all nurses when he comments that 'All men want, not something to do with, but something to do, or rather something to be.' Nurses want to put into practice the nursing values that they have nurtured. They want to nurse because nursing has value for them, and yet it would appear we are in danger of diminishing the value of true nursing by saying that either it can be successfully carried out by others, reducing nursing to a series of observable tasks, or by stating that nursing requires such theoretical and academic preparation that intuition, self-expression and self-fulfilment have little room for movement. Thoreau (1960) notes 'One generation abandons the enterprises of another like stranded vessels' yet perhaps it would be more profitable if we simply re-examined the values of our past and saw what was good and wholesome, what is therefore worth retaining, and what will need to be modified, or abandoned, for we need to heed Thoreau's (1960) note of caution 'beware of all enterprises that require new clothes, and not rather a new maker of clothes.'

It is insufficient to superficially change our ways of behaviour, we must change fundamentally, if we change at all. Thoreau proceeds to say that even though many profess to be learned they are not really so. His comments are addressed to modern academic nurses, if they are addressed to any reader. Thus 'There are nowadays professors of philosophy, but not philosophers. To be a philosopher is not merely to have subtle thoughts, nor even to found a school, but so to love wisdom as to live according to its dictates, a life of simplicity, independence, magnanimity and trust. It is to solve some of the problems of life, not only theoretically, *but practically*' (emphasis mine).

Nurses may not consciously possess specific values, and there may therefore be a problem with the cultivation of specific nursing virtues. However, there definitely are specific attributes and behaviours which are prized by nurses and which nurses seem to hold in esteem (Inglesby, 1992).

In a fascinating book on the analysis of compassion and so-called 'compassionate acts' Wuthnow (1991) approached lay people who were deemed as 'heroic' and asked them to explain how it was that, what to the world appeared to be beyond the call of duty (after all, there is no obligation, to save a child from a burning building) to them seemed the most natural thing to do. Nursing appears to aspire to this type of heroic naturalness, a value so precious it is never actually taught or even spoken of, but like Edith Cavell's shadow weighs heavily on any nurse who cares to stand beneath her statue. Lanara (1988) comments that the values espoused by Henderson (1966) do not come naturally. Before these holistic values can be internalised, it 'requires hard work, practice, continuing learning, evaluation, continuous searching for meaning in her own life. It requires courage, persistence and strength to withstand the failure and frustration that usually accompanies service to other people. It requires heroism' (Lanara, 1988).

Nursing, as any profession, is full of peculiar values, whose collective image approximates nightmares and nonsense more than lofty ideals and dreams of heroism. These oddball values, however, jar against the grain of modern nursing practice. Nursing values appear to be dragged behind the profession's practitioners much as Pooh Bear was dragged behind Christopher

Robin, descending down the stairs, where it was, as far as he knew 'the only way of coming downstairs, but sometimes he feels that there really is another way, if only he could stop bumping for a moment and think of it. And then he feels perhaps there isn't' (Milne, 1951).

References

Abrams, N. (1982). Scope of beneficence in health care. In *Beneficence and Health Care*, E.E. Shelp (ed.), pp. Reidel, London.

Allen, C. (1992). Tradimus. Clause VII. *Nursing Standard*, **6(22)**, 47.

Aristotle (1920). *Poetics*. Translated by I. Bywater. Oxford University Press, Oxford.

Ashworth, P. (1988). Reflections on values. *Intensive Care Nursing*, **4(1)**, 1–2.

Auld, M. (1992). Nurse education past and present. *Nursing Standard*, **6(22)**, 37–9.

Baly, M.E. (1984). *Professional Responsibility*, 2nd edn. Wiley, Chichester.

Browne, J.J. (1992). Uniform feedback. (Letter). *Nursing Times*, **88(14)**, 22.

Carroll, L. (1968). *Alice in Wonderland* and *Through the Looking Glass*. (Minster Classics) Lancer, London.

Davis, G.C. (1988). Nursing values and health care policy. *Nursing Outlook*, **36(6)**, 289–92.

Deremo, D.E. (1989). Integrating professional values, quality practice, productivity and reimbursement for nursing. *Nursing Administration Quarterly*, **14(1)** 9–23

Ellis, P. (1992). The degree nurse debate (Letter). *Nursing Times*, **88(14)**, 23

Farrell, B. (1987). AIDS patients: values in conflict. *Critical Care Nursing Quarterly*, **10(2)**, 74–85.

Fry, S.T. (1986). Moral values and ethical decisions in a constrained economic environment. *Nursing Economics* **4(4)**, 160–4.

Garvin, B.J. and Boyle, K.K. (1985). Values of entering nursing students changes over 10 years. *Research in* Nursing *and Health*, **8(3)**, 235–41

General Nursing Council (GNC) examination papers, 1925 onwards

Glasper, A. and Miller, S. (1992). Newly clothed wards. *Nursing Times*,**88(14)**, 34–6.

Glen, S. (1990). Power for nursing education. *Journal of Advanced Nursing*, **15(11)**, 1335–40.

Hamilton, E. and Cairns, H. (eds) (1961). *The Collected Dialogues of Plato*. (Bollingen series LXXI.) Princetown University Press, Princetown.

Henderson, V. (1966). *The Nature of Nursing*. Macmillan, New York.

Hinkle, D.E., Wiersma, W. and Jurs, S.G. (1982). *Basic Behavioral Statistics* Houghton Mifflin, Boston.

Inglesby, E. (1992). Values and philosophy in nursing: the dynamic of change? In *Nursing: the Challenge to Change*, M. Jolley and G. Brykczynska (eds), pp. 46–70. Edward Arnold, London.

Ives, J.R. (1991). Articulating values and assumptions for strategic planning. *Nursing Management*, **22(1)**, 38–9.

Johnson, M. (1990). Natural sociology and moral questions on nursing: can there be a relationship? *Journal of Advanced Nursing*, **15(12)**, 1358–62.

Jolley, M. (1989). The professionalization of nursing: the uncertain path. In *Current Issues in Nursing*, Jolley M and Allen P (eds). Jolley and P. Allan (eds), pp. 1–22 Chapman & Hall, London.

Kelly, B. (1991). The professional values of English nursing undergraduates. *Journal of Advanced Nursing*, **16(7)**, 867–72.

Kelman, H. (1966). Three processes of social influence. In *Attitudes: Selected Readings*, M. Jahoda and N. Warren (Eds). Penguin, Harmondsworth.

King, I.M. (1971). *Toward a Theory of Nursing*. Wiley, New York.

Kingsley, C. (1986). *The Water Babies*. Puffin, Harmondsworth.

Kohlberg, L. (1969). A cognitive development approach to socialization. In *Handbook of Socialization*, D. Goslin (ed.). Rand MacNally, Chicago.

Kopelman, L. (1984). Respect and the retarded: issues of valuing and labeling. In *Ethics and Mental Retardation*, L. Kopelman and P.J.C. Mosko (eds). Reidel, Dordrecht.

Kramer, M. (1974). *Reality Shock*. Mosby, St Louis.

Lanara, V.A. (1988). Cultural values – influence on the delivery of care. Intensive *Care Nursing*, **4(1)**, 3–8.

Leininger, M. (1978). *Transcultural Nursing: Concepts, Theories and Practices* Wiley, New York.

Lockley, P. (1992). Points of view. *Nursing Standard*, **6(22)**, 43.

Long, I. (1992). 'To protect the public and ensure justice is done': an examination fo the Philip Donnelly case. *Journal of Advanced Nursing*, **17(1)**, 5–9.

Matthew, A. (1992). The degree nurse debate (Letter). *Nursing Times*, **88(14)**, 23.

Milne, A.A. (1952). *Winnie-the-Pooh*. Methuen, London.

Murdoch, I. (1970). *Sovereignty of Good*. Routledge & Kegan Paul, London.

Nagel, T. (1980). The limits of objectivity. In *The Tanner Lectures on Human Values. Volume One*, S. McMurrin (ed.), University of Utah Press, Salt Lake City.

Omery, A. (1989). Values, moral reasoning and ethics. *Nursing Clinics of North America*, **24(2)**, 499–508.

Plume, A. (1988). *Sister Plume's Notes on Nursing: a Collection of Letters to the Editor of the Nursing Times*. Macmillan, Basingstoke.

Raths, L.E., Harmin, M. and Simon, S.B. (1978). *Values and Teaching*, 2nd edn. Merrill, Columbus.

Raya, A. (1990). Can knowledge be promoted and values ignored? Implications for nursing education. *Journal of Advanced Nursing*, **15(5)**, 504–9.

Reilly, D.E. (1989). Ethics and values in nursing: are we opening Pandora's box? *Nursing and Health Care*, **10(2)**, 91–5.

Rokeach, M. (1973). *The Nature of Human Values*. Free Press, New York.

Rosenhand, L. (1973). On being Sane in insane places. *Science*, **179**, 250–8.

Sellar, W.C. and Yeatman, R.J. (1930). *1066 and All That*. Magnet, London.

Shorter Oxford English Dictionary (1973). *Volume 2*, 3rd edn. Clarendon, Oxford.

Silver, M. (1976). *Values Education*. National Education Association, Washington, DC.

Smith, M.J. (1990). Caring: ubiquitous or unique. *Nursing Science Quarterly*, **3(2)**, 54.

Sparrow, S. (1991). An exploration of the role of the nurse's uniform through a period of non-uniform wear on an acute medical ward. *Journal of Advanced Nursing*, **16(1)**, 116–22.

Steele, S.M. (1986). AIDS: clarifying values to close in on ethical questions. *Nursing and Health Care*, **7(5)**, 247–8.

Thompson, J.E. and Thompson, H.O. (1990). Values: directional signals for life choices. *Neonatal Network*, **8(4)**, 83–94.

Thoreau, H.D. (1960). *Walden AND On the Duty of Civil Disobedience*. Signet Classics, New York.

Uustal, D.B. (1987). Values: the cornerstone of nursing's moral art. In *Ethics at the Bedside*, M.D. Fowler and Levine-Ariff, J. (eds). Lippincott, Philadelphia, pp. 136–70.

Wright, J. (1992). Bringing back the cap (Letter). *Nursing Times*, **88(7)**, 16.

Williams, B. (1981). *Moral Luck: Philosophical Papers 1973–1980*. Cambridge University Press, Cambridge.

Wuthnow, R. (1991). *Acts of Compassion: Caring for Others and Helping Ourselves*. Princeton University Press, Princetown.

7 Closing thoughts on hidden agendas – an epilogue

This book has explored aspects of the nature of nursing, focusing on those issues which the authors believe constitute its 'hidden agendas': in the values which have historically shaped it and which currently influence it; in the psychological processes whereby those values are transmitted and acquired; in the sociological factors and political processes which affect the content and context of nursing; and in the education which inspires and enables, or constrains and inhibits, students as they learn the art and science of nursing. These hidden agendas operate below the surface of explicit recognition, and sometimes even below the conscious awareness of nurses and those influencing nursing.

This final chapter offers some additional suggestions of 'hidden agendas' not covered by previous authors, and concludes on a positive note, identifying 'overt agendas' and emphasising that the future of nursing can be shaped by nurses in ways which not only enhance nursing's distinctive contribution to health care, for the benefit of nurses, but most importantly, for the benefit of those whom it is nursing's privilege to serve: patients and clients; their families and communities; the society in which we live and work; and the international community.

It is in the nature of hidden agendas that they may be uncomfortable and challenging. Some of the issues we might be reluctant to address may include developments in nursing education and practice which stemmed from reasonable reactions to previous problems, but where the pendulum of reform has swung too far, creating new problems. But as initiating change requires commitment, and innovation demands courage and hard endeavour, those who have worked to bring in changes are often understandably reluctant to admit the limitations of their achievements. Thus reforms tend to become entrenched and reformers may become conservative and resistant to further reform – creating new 'hidden agendas' to preserve their own new status quo. The following list identifies some additional hidden, as well as overt, agendas currently relevant within the context of nursing care.

Additional hidden agendas

1. Definitions of nursing: status versus service?
2. The move away from the 'medical model' in nurse education – enhancement or betrayal of nursing?
3. Politics and policy-making: contribution or confusion?
4. Changing health needs in the global village: challenge and opportunity.

Overt agendas

1. Values of nursing: compassion and skilled companionship;
2. Nursing education: teleological criteria;
3. Professionalism and politics in partnership;
4. Nursing's distinctive contribution to health care internationally.

Hidden agendas in nursing values: status versus service?

Much of the discussion in earlier chapters has focused on the values underpinning nursing and the extent to which they inhibit or enhance nursing's status and its position in power structures. These are important considerations, as they influence the extent to which nurses are able to exert pressure, not only for their own benefit, but also for the benefit of those whom they serve. Much of the emphasis in health policy has traditionally been on medical priorities, with a preference in resource allocation on cure rather than care. In many ways this is understandable on a rational basis, and is not necessarily the result of a sinister conspiracy or abuse of power, as is sometimes implied. Who would not prefer cure to care?

However, there are many situations where people do need care and where they suffer from conditions for which there is no cure. Traditionally, these are the 'Cinderella' situations which tend to be less generously resourced, and where vulnerable people may suffer from inadequate provision. And there may be power politics at work in the distribution of influence in key decision-making arenas, especially those which hold the purse-strings.

This makes it all the more important that nurses act as advocates and make the case publicly for the funding necessary for good quality care. Nurses must also make the case for the value of nursing and its distinctive contribution to health care. In so doing, they should articulate clearly the key values which underpin nursing. These are quintessentially timeless and, in their distinctiveness, should be affirmed as indispensable, unique, valuable and valued. Two of these key values are encapsulated in words which share the Latin prefix 'com': compassion and companionship. They both emphasise the special characteristics of nursing: 'compassion', which is to *be with* those in need, in their suffering; and 'companionship', which means literally to share bread, but symbolises the role of the nurse in helping another person with intimate, basic, personal needs.

Of course, compassion and companionship are not unique to nursing. Other caring professions identify with those who suffer and so share their suffering with them. But nurses, in the intimacy and round-the-clock personal care they provide, embody these values of compassion and companionship in a special and distinctive way. This is highlighted in the concept of 'skilled companionship', which is identified by Alastair Campbell as nursing's unique and valuable contribution among the caring professions.

> A way of understanding the 'loving as caring' which is required in nursing may be found by exploring the concept of companionship . . . The skill of companionship lies in sensing the need of the other person and accommodating oneself to the other's idiosyncrasies. Skilled

nursing care depends upon such sensitivity . . . Secondly, nursing is a companionship which helps the person onward. Whether the destination is recovery or death a companion helps the hardness of the journey. So the good companion looks ahead and encourages when all seems lost. The skill and knowledge of nurses makes them able to see, often better than the patient, how the journey can be accomplished . . . Thirdly, the closeness of contact between nurse and patient means a costly mutuality for the nurse. It involves 'being with' not just 'doing to' . . . Finally, the commitment of companionship is a limited one . . . Although it can be painful, parting is an essential element of companionship. The other person journeys on – to life or death. Thus in the skilled care which the professional nurse offers there may be discerned a form of love.

(Campbell, 1984; pp. 49–51)

This concept of skilled companionship provides a constellation of values which can provide criteria for judging some of the contentious issues confronting nursing today and preoccupying nurses, sometimes with destructive conflict. For example, the issue addressed earlier, as to whether nurses should wear uniform, should be resolved according to the principle of 'whatever is best for patients, or clients'. If *they* feel more happy with staff in clearly identifiable uniforms (as may be the case with some people in highly dependent conditions) then that should count more than nurses' personal preferences; if, however, paediatric nurses find that children are happier with nurses in different kinds of attire, then the children's well-being should be the deciding factor. This is one of many issues which could be decided by research, on a flexible basis, centred on patients' and clients' needs and wishes. All the status-conscious obsessions about the historical characteristics of uniforms derived from a Victorian age, associated with the concept of servitude, are nowhere near as important as the extent to which a patient in intensive care, or a frail elderly resident in continuing care, feels happier and more confident with staff in uniform or in mufti.

A commitment to research is one of the most fundamental values which should underpin nursing. For it is only by knowledge derived from research that we can be sure that our practice is as effective as possible. Otherwise, the only basis for practice must be part of an unholy trinity: untested tradition; unjustified prejudice or irrational dogma. Tradition may be good, but we need to test its effectiveness; prejudice may be justifiable, but we must be prepared to justify it; dogma may be sound, but we must be ready to demonstrate its validity. Too often, in nursing, we have done things in certain ways, because 'Sister (or some other authority figure) always likes it done this way' or 'This is how it has always been done'.

Research in nursing practice in the United Kingdom has indicated that too often procedures and practices may be based on the unholy trinity, rather than on scientific assessment of effectiveness. For example, the survey undertaken by the Nursing Practice Research Unit (1983) on the treatment of pressure sores found an enormous variety of procedures in different hospitals, some of which were very strange! Such diversity of practice indicates that treatments cannot have been based on rigorous scientific analysis of care-effectiveness or cost-effectiveness. This finding has serious implications, most importantly in terms of human suffering, but also in terms of financial costs.

It was perhaps this commitment to research, to ensure that nursing care was of the highest quality, which prompted the famous dictum attributed to Florence Nightingale, 'To understand God's thoughts, we must study statistics, for these are the measure of His purpose.'

The move away from the 'medical model' in nurse education – enhancement or betrayal of nursing?

The move towards an education for nurses which is truly 'education' and not just 'training' is a development to be warmly welcomed and encouraged. The progress from being taught 'How', to being encouraged also to think and to ask 'Why', is essential for safe, sensitive and competent professional practice.

A personal anecdote illustrates the extent to which the culture of nursing has progressed over 30 years. I will never forget my first ward report. The ward sister was someone for whom I had profound admiration: clinically superb; sensitive with patients and their relatives; an inspiring teacher for students – an excellent role model. I was relieved to receive a good report, especially as I had such respect for her. Then, as I was turning to leave her office, she called me back with these final words: 'Just one word of advice, nurse: as you go through the hospital, please, for your own sake, do not ask so many awkward questions.'

I was a very shy 18-year-old, and I could not remember asking any questions, let alone awkward ones. But such was the culture of hospitals in general, and nursing in particular, that this dedicated ward sister believed I would make myself unpopular if I dared to question anything. Therefore, recent developments such as Project 2000 are vitally important. They should enable students to have time to reflect on knowledge and practice; to learn theory before its application; to acquire a broader base of disciplines; and to develop a research-orientation which should engender a life-long critical approach to ensure that care given is of the highest possible standard.

However, there are some hidden agendas deeply rooted in current educational theories and practices which may not be very conducive to safe, competent practice. For example, as nurse education has moved into institutions of higher and further education, there has been a tendency in some places for nurses to undervalue nursing and to sell the nursing input cheap. This is totally unnecessary. What nursing has to offer is immensely valuable; not only in crude terms of resources, although they are important. But more important are high quality students, well motivated, dedicated to service, and bringing rich experience from the clinical field into university and college classrooms.

However, some non-nursing academic staff in some institutions of higher and further education have had their own agendas and sought to impose their own subjects without adequate adjustment to the interests and needs of nursing students, and at the expense of subjects needed by nursing students. This has been the case particularly with social scientists, who tend to predominate in the faculties in which nursing is located, who have sometimes imposed social sciences onto the curriculum at the expense of clinical sciences.

In some cases, nurse educators have opposed this shift away from adequate coverage of clinical sciences. But in other situations, this shift has coincided with a tendency for nurse educators themselves to wish to dissociate from the 'medical model' in nurse education. This has positive and negative implications. For example, it may reflect positive changes in attitudes and values in nursing care, moving from a predominantly disease-oriented approach to a more humanistic and holistic appreciation of patients as people with spiritual, psychological, social and physical needs. Student nurses are less likely now to talk (and hence to think) about patients, as happened in earlier days, as 'the coronary in the fourth bed on the left'.

So far, so good. But the pendulum has perhaps swung too far when some new pre-registration courses for Project 2000 or nursing degree qualifications, pare down clinical science to levels which raise questions about adequate knowledge bases for safe practice. As Chairman of the Health Studies Committee of the Council for National Academic Awards, I had the privilege of participating in validating procedures for many new courses, some of them excellent. But on too many occasions, I and my colleagues were concerned by the inadequacy of clinical science teaching. For example, one proposed degree course contained no pharmacology and virtually no pathology (even with 'non-medical' names). The proposed justification for these omissions was the rationale that this was a degree in nursing, concentrating on 'health' – health promotion and health education. When the validating panel expressed concern over the lack of any reference to key nursing responsibilities, such as the care of an unconscious patient, the reply was that this would be covered under the topic of 'mobility'.

This is an extreme example of an abreaction from the 'medical model'. But other examples were also cause for concern, as with another proposed course which only allowed 'nursing' and biological sciences just over one tenth of the first and second year studies, the rest being social and behavioural sciences of various kinds. As students could qualify with the Project 2000 Diploma at the end of the second year, this minute proportion of time spent on what might reasonably be deemed knowledge necessary for safe practice, seemed grossly inadequate.

While appreciating that health promotion is a welcome addition to nursing's remit, and behavioural sciences are an important part of nurse education, such a massive swing of the pendulum away from the 'medical model' as represented by clinical sciences must raise serious questions. For the main part of the responsibilities associated with most aspects of general nursing will always surely, inevitably, be to assist people who are ill, injured, frail or otherwise incapacitated, with their activities of daily living, which they are unable to perform for themselves; and to co-operate with medical and other colleagues in therapies necessary for the recovery of health or the alleviation of suffering. To jettison the scientific knowledge base for clinical practice in a hidden agenda in pursuit of a 'non-medical' role for nursing is to risk betraying the raison d'être of nursing and those for whom nursing is professionally responsible.

There has also been a shift in attitudes to the assessment of clinical competence with the move, now long-established, away from the task-oriented approach reflected in the old 'procedure books' to just four ward-based clinical assessments, two of which involved no 'hands-on care' at all.

This shift away from the systematic assessment of practical clinical competences, which resulted in the jettisoning of traditional 'procedure books' (usually of certain colours – ours was the 'blue book') also led to the jettisoning of almost every kind of systematic clinical supervision and assessment. Was the hidden agenda the insecurity of educators confronting their own lack of contact with, and confidence in, the real world of clinical practice?

During non-participant observation undertaken as part of a research project on student nurses' clinical learning (Jacka and Lewin, 1987), I and my colleagues witnessed some of the results of this swing of the pendulum, with numerous examples of serious deficiencies in the quality of care given to patients, and of unsuitable demands put on students. One typical illustration must suffice. A second year student who had completed the assessment for aseptic technique during her first year, was asked to remove a drain from a large incision in a man's neck; she had never undertaken such a procedure before, but was deemed competent to do so. In the process, she failed to notice that the tubing was secured by a safety pin on the other side of the patient's neck. A non-participant researcher who happened to be observing quickly shed the 'non-participant' role! It was not the student who was to blame, but the system which allowed students to be given responsibilities without the insurance policy of the procedure book which enabled the nurse in charge to see at a glance exactly which nursing responsibilities students had mastered and those for which they needed support and supervision.

This research also indicated the extremely patchy nature of the clinical experiences and competences acquired by students as they passed through their clinical learning areas. As they came up to final examinations and anticipated emerging as qualified staff, many of them were deeply apprehensive of taking responsibility on wards, knowing their lacunae in assessed hands-on care.

Nursing education should not suffer from these hidden agendas. For, like all professional education, its overt agendas should rest on explicit, clearly formulated, comprehensive *teleological criteria*. In other words, the curriculum, including a curriculum of clinical competence, and all forms of assessment should be judged by the extent to which they ensure that practitioners are adequately prepared to fulfil the responsibilities required of them once they are qualified, and to do so safely, competently and sensitively, in ways which respect the integrity of those for whom they care.

Politics and policy-making: contribution or confusion?

Trevor Clay in his book 'Nurses: Power and Politics' has made a strong case for nurses to become more involved in politics, reflecting some of the themes in Chapter 6. He claims: 'Politics, power and nursing are part of the same fabric. The profession cannot separate them.'
and he concludes:

I hope that other nurses will, like me, see political participation as clean and positive and not dirty and negative. Each day we spend working with people we see their needs and the services they deserve. We must look beyond the immediate frustration of not being able to give all we could for today's patients but resolve, as individuals, as I believe is our duty, to do everything reasonable within our power and through our nursing organisations to make sure that tomorrow's people get the nurses and nursing they deserve. I am confident that together we can be a powerhouse for change (p.151).

It is vital for nurses as members of a caring profession to become involved directly or indirectly in the political arena, if we are to fulfil our advocacy role. Many nurses are reluctant to engage in discussions on politics and policy-making, often reflecting hidden agendas of unwillingness to become associated with any controversy and of 'not wanting to get involved'. But advocacy is a part of nursing's responsibilities. Nurses are in the front line; there is no-one better placed to assess and to evaluate the effects of laws and policies on those in need.

This is a time of radical change in all countries, with changing patterns of morbidity, mortality and the provision of health care. There is thus an urgent need for systematic monitoring, research and reporting to evaluate changing health needs and to publicise the effects of health and welfare policies. They must be systematically and impartially tried and tested: if they are successful, then it is important to document the success to build on good practice; if there are unforeseen problems, it is important to identify them quickly in order to take corrective action. For in the field of health and welfare, problems may cause real suffering, and often that suffering is found among the most vulnerable people, least able to articulate their needs or assert their rights.

This danger of negative unforeseen effects of health and welfare policies is associated with the inevitable fact that in health care, every success in prevention or cure becomes, in turn, a new challenge. In Western societies, this century is unsurpassed in human history in the dramatic growth in knowledge and practice which has resulted in annihilation of many killer diseases, the ability to treat effectively many conditions which cannot be prevented, with a consequent increase in both length and quality of life for the majority of people which would have been inconceivable only a few decades ago.

With these advances however have come new problems, challenges and hidden agendas. For example, the challenges of caring for children suffering from infectious diseases, in Western countries now relegated to history books, have been replaced by the challenges of providing for the growing numbers of frail and infirm elderly people, with care which respects their dignity and maximises their quality of life. The major exception to the general pattern of increased life expectancy is the tragic advent of AIDS. But, in very general terms, the problems now confronting health care in Western societies have shifted qualitatively, causing new challenges, especially the challenge of agonising choice between competing priorities.

In the past, when often there was no remedy, in the form of prevention or cure, choice was limited or non-existent. But where potential remedies abound, policy decisions must be made, which often involve hidden agendas concerning power and money, as well as profound ethical problems. These problems arise at the 'macro', or societal level, such as choice in expenditure of finite resources: on prevention or cure, or on institutional or community care. They also arise at the 'micro' level, concerning individual patients or clients and their families. For example, as knowledge and technology make extension of life possible, they also require decisions when to end it, with all the resulting ethical dilemmas surrounding the management of death. Many of these ethical dilemmas are inevitably associated with individuals' own deepest beliefs and values, potentially influencing hidden agendas relating to attitudes and practices concerning life and death – and the management of death. Very soon, there is likely to be public debate and political decisions on such key issues as euthanasia and 'living wills'. What will be nursing's contribution to these debates? And how will each individual nurse resolve these dilemmas in his or her own practice? Hidden agendas and covert policies may have to become open and public, with all the ethical and professional challenges which will inevitably be involved.

But these challenges reflect developments in health needs and health care which also provide ever-unfolding opportunities. For example, in the care of the elderly, new and exciting initiatives have been established, such as the Nursing Development Units based on nursing rather then medical needs, allowing more individualised care, especially for the long-stay frail elderly; and the application of primary nursing in various settings (see Wright, 1990). In the care of the dying, there has been the extension of the hospice movement, where staff strive to enable the dying and their families to experience death as a meaningful part of life.

Recent reforms in the National Health Service (NHS) have not been without their problems, as highlighted in previous chapters. But they also create opportunities which can involve nurses and their creative potential in shaping significant developments. For example, in West Lambeth Community Care (NHS) Trust, the Chief Executive is a nurse and some initiatives reflect a distinctively nursing approach to the provision of care – such as night respite care for confused elderly people. This allows families to have a good night's sleep, and enables them to continue to care for their elderly relative at home, without having to endure the pain of requesting admission to residential care because of the impossibility of providing adequate night care. This policy is both care-effective and cost-effective and is an example of a nursing initiative stemming from a positive, creative approach to the health challenges confronting contemporary society.

The development of community care has enabled many previously institutionalised patients to find new dignity and independence as citizens of the wider community. But community care is another arena where hidden agendas may be operative in ways adversely affecting patients, clients and their families. For example, the National Health Service and Community Care Act delegates primary responsibility for community care to the social service departments of local authorities. If some politically motivated authorities allow hidden agendas to influence their policies and provisions, this could be a recipe for potential disaster for some of their most vulnerable citizens – the elderly, the mentally ill and mentally handicapped

For example, the Act makes it possible for social service departments to ignore the contribution of health professionals in the assessment of the needs of their clients. Examples are already coming to light of problems of lack of co-operation in this vital process. And some local authorities could use vulnerable groups as political canon-fodder, failing, for example, to provide essential supplies such as incontinence pads for the elderly, in order to blame central government for inadequate funding. Examples of these tactics are also already coming to light. The tragedy is that the client groups who will suffer most are those least able to assert their rights or to articulate their needs.

These are further examples of success creating the potential for new problems. The concept of community care was based on humane and idealistic motives. But its implementation may be fraught with problems. This scenario highlights yet again the fundamental need for continuing research to monitor the effects of political policies. No-one is better placed to do this than nurses at the frontline of care. As Dr Mahler of The World Health Organisation emphasised in a keynote address in 1987 entitled 'Leadership in Nursing in Health For All':

> Nurses have always had a strong dedication and commitment to social causes and have shown an acceptance of and a readiness to change. They provide care at all levels and in all settings which gives them direct contact with the population. They are frequently the main link between individuals, the family and the rest of the health system and they form the largest sector of health workers in many countries . . . They are eminently positioned to voice the feelings of the people whom they serve and to give them credibility and reasoned support and are often seen as natural leaders at the community level.
>
> (WHO, 1987)

This brings us back to the issue of nursing's involvement in politics. It is important that political activity by nurses must be imbued with professional ethics and a compassionate concern for those for whom nursing is professionally responsible. In so far as we are motivated by the ideals of service, rather than by self-interest and status, we are likely to command respect and support. To paraphrase a former President of the International Council of Nurses, Madam Laballe: nurses have a great and indisputable moral advantage. In so far as we are the patient's or the community's advocate, our endeavours are essentially altruistic. If our political activities are not primarily motivated by professional self-interest but by the common good, they command respect. This should enable us to fulfil our responsibilities as the major caring profession by using our political influence and leadership potential on behalf of those we serve.

Over twenty centuries ago in ancient Athens, Pericles, the famous orator and advocate of the world's earliest democracy, made a similar point. Challenging the citizens of Athens to take a responsible part in public affairs, he claimed: 'We do not say that a person who takes no interest in politics is minding his own business; rather, we say he has no business here at all' (Thucydides, 1972; p. 147).

This challenge, echoing down over two thousand years, reflects a basic principle which links the worlds of the professional and the politician. It is a principle which should apply to all politicians, and also to all professionals and educators: a commitment to having open ears, open eyes and an open mind before having an open mouth.

We must all be willing to look, to listen, and to learn, and to try to acknowledge our own hidden agendas. And we must be prepared to listen to criticism, and to rethink our ideas and practices where they are shown to be inadequate or inappropriate. This principle has been expounded convincingly in many works on the philosophy of science and on social reform, especially those written by Karl Popper (1945 and 1963) in which he analyses the essentially tentative nature of scientific knowledge and the need for a perpetually humble and critical approach to social reforms.

Changing health needs in the global village: challenge and opportunity

There is an ancient Chinese curse: 'May you live in interesting times.' For anyone with an interest in Health Care, there can scarcely be a more interesting time in which to live than the present. It is a time of challenge, change and opportunity, although some of the challenges appear so daunting and so tragic that they may feel like curses.

One of the results of preoccupation with hidden agendas in our own society is that they tend to cause introspective concern and to lead to neglect of problems and challenges elsewhere in our global village.

Therefore, before the book concludes, it is important to look briefly at wider horizons and the challenges, changes and opportunities confronting us in the Second and Third worlds respectively. Because their health needs and the corresponding challenges vary so fundamentally, it is impossible to generalise. Illustrative examples must serve as indicators of need and challenges for response.

In the Second World of eastern and central Europe and the former Soviet Union, the challenges are formidable. Now that the Iron Curtain has come down, there are much greater opportunities to learn about health challenges and ways in which we may work with professional colleagues in those previously isolated countries. For example, Poland suffered devastation of its health care system during the dark years of martial law in the 1980s. The hidden agenda of the Communist government was the destruction of the morale and resistance of the Polish people, who were opposing Communist ideology and Soviet influence. Consequently, the health care system was deprived of virtually everything: in many places, there were no essential supplies such as bandages; often there were no medicines; in one intensive care unit, the drug cupboard was empty, except for vitamin C. Basic nursing supplies such as incontinence pads were non-existent; there were no disinfectants or soap. Essential therapies were totally inadequate: for example, children with treatable leukaemias died as doctors, nurses and parents watched helplessly and hopelessly. Yet the quality of medical and nursing care was remarkably high, because, as the director of one hospital put it: 'Staff give of themselves to make up for what they haven't got.'

Economic catastrophe and environmental disaster have left behind a lethal legacy. For example, in the late 1980s, the national figure for life expectancy for men had fallen by five years in five years, from 69–64; and in Southern Poland, only 3 per cent of men were living to receive their pension at the age of 65. At the other end of the life-span, the infant mortality rate was rising. In the old university city of Cracow, researchers found no normal placentas in mothers recently giving birth in the nearby steel city of Nova Huta.

Now the people of Poland breathe the air of freedom, even if much of it is still environmentally polluted. They are keen to improve their health care. They greatly value help, especially exchanges, as they have been isolated for so many decades from developments in the rest of the world. We have much to learn from them and much to share with them.

In Russia, children are still suffering from one of the hidden agendas of the former Soviet system. Many children are taken into the care of the state, following domestic problems of broken homes, alcoholism, overcrowding and acute poverty. At a Conference on Human Rights in Leningrad in 1990, two of the newly democratically elected City Councillors (Deputies) highlighted a disturbing tendency to classify many of these children coming into care as mentally handicapped or 'oligophrenics', even when they appeared to be of average or above average intellectual ability. Once classified as 'oligophrenic', they were denied a proper education; choice of a job; the opportunity for family life and other basic human rights. They were thus condemned to tragically stunted lives and virtual slave labour. The City Deputies who had courageously drawn attention to this policy identified the hidden agenda as the use by the state of these children to satisfy its need for 'unthinking manual workers'. The Deputies were keen to try to remedy this exploitation of children and the violation of their basic human rights. They therefore asked for help in establishing independent data, based on internationally accepted norms, to help them to challenge and to change the policy. A multidisciplinary team from Britain returned, at the request of these Russians, to assess some of the children. The findings are reported in the report *Trajectories of Despair* (Cox, 1991). The team assessed 171 children in 15 orphanages of so-called 'oligophrenics' in Moscow and St Petersburg and found that two thirds of them were of average or above average ability. This research has since led to various positive initiatives, such as exchanges of personnel and the establishment of new orphanages and homes for street children in Moscow and St Petersburg.

The Third World poses different challenges. For example, many places face the ultimate tragedy of vast numbers of people suffering and dying from avoidable diseases. Countries like Sudan face a double dimension of tragedy: man-made catastrophe superimposed on natural disasters such as drought, flood and famine. There are an estimated five million displaced people forced off their homelands by conflict and the threat of massacre. Hundreds of thousands of refugees are in camps, with virtually nothing; and especially in the South, under attack by forces from the government in the North, there is a desperate shortage of food and medical supplies. For example, one hospital serves a catchment area of 700,000 people, with virtually nothing – no electricity, running water or adequate medical supplies.

The final example is a place generally acknowledged as one of the worst hell-holes in the contemporary world: Nagorno Karabakh, the small Armenian enclave cruelly located by Stalin within Azerbaijan. Blockaded, bombarded, besieged by the government of Azerbaijan, the Armenian inhabitants there also have virtually nothing. In January 1992, casualties with amputations, burns, glass in eyes, had no anaesthetics or analgesics; civilians in towns and villages have been deprived of fuel, electricity, running water, adequate medicines and basic food, including milk and baby milk powder. Major aid organisations could not gain access, because the territory is officially part of Azerbaijan, and the government of Azerbaijan, with a hidden agenda of ethnic cleansing, delayed or denied permission for access. Consequently, United Nations organisations have been unable to help and the International Committee of the Red Cross could not gain access until April 1992. Their help has been limited by logistical problems and the continuing Azeri offensive. Therefore there has been a critical vacuum in provision of desperately needed aid, only met by organisations committed to putting humanitarian need before political constraints – such as Medecins Sans Frontieres and Christian Solidarity International.

This tragic situation raises a final example of challenge and opportunity for response. There is a growing need for relief and health programmes in such countries. There is also a need for a United Kingdom rapid relief task force – something which is surprisingly missing in this country. The time is ripe for the development of a United Kingdom organisation like Medecins Sans Frontieres. This country is especially well placed to develop this, with some of the best nursing expertise in the world, and with a well-grounded national tradition of voluntary work.

The need for such rapid relief response will unfortunately grow in the years ahead. Natural disasters are inevitable. But also, tragically, the number of areas throughout the world where brutal regimes inflict repression and death on vulnerable minorities appears to be increasing, especially with the breaking up of the former Soviet Empire. Thus, there is a likelihood of an ever-growing number of conflicts like those in former Yugoslavia, Sudan and Nagorno Karabakh.

The motto of the Royal London Hospital, is 'Humani Nihil a Me Alienum Puto'. It can be translated as 'My concern must be for all humanity.' It is a salutary reminder that one of nursing's most fundamental values must be a commitment to help all citizens in need in our global village, regardless of colour, race, creed or location. There is no more urgent time for the application of this ideal. We now live in a world where that desirable goal of 'Health for All by 2000' seems to be receding rather than approaching. Millions of people suffer in situations where they could be helped. For them, many must feel that these 'interesting days' are indeed cursed.

I hope that this book, uncovering some of the hidden agendas which have inhibited nursing and nurses from making their full potential contribution to health care, will also stimulate new and positive initiatives, so that the interesting times in which we live, do not become a curse, but a time of creative responses to the changes, challenges and opportunities which confront us all.

This chapter has tried to indicate that nursing is in a powerful position to influence not only the future of nursing itself, but the provision of health care in this country and abroad. These words of Sir William Osler apply as much to nurses today as they did to the physicians to whom he addressed them nearly a century ago:

> Tis no idle challenge which we throw out to the world when we claim that our mission is of the highest and of the noblest kind, not alone in curing disease but in educating the people in the laws of health and in preventing the spread of plagues and pestilences . . . Not that we can all live up to the highest ideals . . . far from it – we are only human. But we have ideals, which means much, and they are realizable, which means more . . .
>
> (Strauss, 1968; p. 409)

If we endeavour to live up to our highest professional values, and to fight for them in the policy-making arenas, we can develop agendas which will help to make our profession more care-effective and our world more humane. The opportunities are vast, the need is urgent and the time is now.

References

Campbell, A.V. (1984). *Moderated Love: a Theology of Professional Care*. SPCK, London.

Cox, C. (1991). *Trajectories of Despair: Misclassification and Maltreatment* of Soviet Orphans. Christian Solidarity International, Zurich.

Clay, T. (1987). *Nurses: Power and Politics*. Heinemann, London.

David, J.A., Chapman, R.G., Chapman, E.J., and Lockett, B. (1983). *An Investigation of the Current Methods Used in Nursing for the Care of Patients with Established Pressure Sores*. Northwick Park Hospital Nursing Practice Research Unit, Harrow.

Jacka, K. and Lewin, D. (1987). *The Clinical Learning of Student Nurses*. King's College, University of London Nursing Education Research Unit, London.

Popper, K. (1945). *The Open Society and Its Enemies*. Routledge and Kegan Paul, London.

Popper K. (1963). *Conjectures and Refutations*. Routledge and Kegan Paul, London.

Strauss, M.B. (ed.) (1968). *Familiar Medical Quotations*, Churchill, London.

Thucydides (1972). *History of the Peloponnesian War*, Penguin, Harmondsworth.

World Health Organisation (WHO) (1987). *Leadership for health for all The challenge to Nursing. A strategy for action*. British Life Assurance Trust for Health and Medical, Education, London.

WRIGHT, S.G. (1990). *My Patient – My Nurse: the Practice of Primary Nursing*. Scutari, London.

Index

Attitudes
  consistency theories 25
  definitions 22
  development 24–6
  educational influence 34–6
  functional approach 26
  holders of 23
  inconsistent 25, 34
  schema of 24–5
  social cognition and 30–1
  structural approach 21–5
  values and 23–4, 135
Attitudes, change of
  Congruity Theory 25
  factors influencing 26–7
Attitudes, transmission
  attribution theory 28–30
  social learning theory 27–8
  socialisation and 32–4
Attribution theory 28–30
Attributions
  actor (observer) error 30
  external (situational) 29
  false consensus effect 30
  fundamental attribution error 29
  internal (personal) 29

Behaviour, attribution theory 28–30
Beliefs, definition 22
Buildings 99
Bullying at work 52
Bureaucracy
  and educational structures 99–100
  and nurses 62–3, 74–5
  and patient care 63
  and status of health professionals 71

Care/caring 160–1
  as foundation of education 102–3
  mentality of 47, 63
  role of nurses 45–6, 48, 56–63
  valuing of 68–9, 72–3, 76
  see also community care; health care
Chadwick, Edwin 3

Code of Conduct (UKCC) 126
Cognition, social 30–1
Cognitive dissonance 25, 27, 32
Community care 166–7
Companionship 160–1
Compassion 160–1
Concealment, use in work control 53–5
Curriculum 84–9, 149, 151, 162–4
Curriculum, hidden
  acting on 101–2
  definitions 80–2
  finding 101
  messages and strategies 83–4
  nursing 27, 82, 84–9, 92–103
  pupil labelling 89–90
  racial discrimination 91–5
  theoretical perspectives 100–1
  timetabling 84–6

Discrimination 91–5, 113–14
Dissonance, cognitive 25, 27, 32

Eastern Europe, health needs 168–9
Economics
  Project 2000 114–16
  remuneration 118–19
Education of nurses
  assessment in 94–6
  curriculum 84–9, 149, 151, 162–4
  discrimination in 92–5
  English National Board Higher
    Award 35
  ethnic minorities 94–6
  examination topics 147–9
  funding 114–16
  hidden curriculum see curriculum,
    hidden
  influence on attitudes 34–6
  language use in 89
  nurse educators in 36–8
  organisational structures 99–100
  politics of 114–17
  Post Registration Education and
    Practice Project (PREPP) 35

Project 2000 35, 36–7, 114, 163
  resources 98–9
  student coping strategies 86–9
  theory and practice in 35–6, 149–55,
    162–4
  timetables 84–6
  values in 144–9, 163
  see also students; teachers
Elderly, care of 165–6
Ethnic minorities in nursing 94–6,
  113–14

Feminism 16–17
  liberal 16
  Marxist approach 16
  and nursing 17
  radical 16–17
  socialist 16
  Victorian era 9–10, 16
Free speech, suppression 54

Gender
  of health care workers 69–71
  and status of nurses 66–7
Grading, clinical 118–19

Health care
  global challenges 168–70
  politics of 123–4, 127, 160, 165–7
Health care support workers (HCSW)
  117–18

Images of nurses/nursing 112–13
  media and 121–3
Industrial action 108, 120–1
Information processing
  levels of 25
  schemas 24–5
Institutions *see* organisations/institutions
Integration group 34

Labelling of students 89–90
  racial 91–5
Language, use of 89, 153–4
Learning
  assessment 97–8
  latent 28
  social 27–8, 66
  see also education: students
Library facilities 98–9

Management
  health service 75–6
  nursing 74–5

Managers, nursing 71
Media and nurses/training 112, 121–3
Mistakes, attitude to 146
Models of nursing 152–3

Nagorno Karabakh, health needs 170
National Health Service reforms 123–4,
  127, 154, 166
Needs hierarchies 32
  prejudices in 66
Nightingale, Florence 10–11, 140
  nurse training 11–12, 15–16
  nursing reforms 11–12, 15
  view of nurses 12–13
Nurse educators *see* teachers
Nurse managers 71
Nurses
  political 108, 127–8
  Victorian 10, 12–15
Nursing
  historical background 1–10
  and medicine 69
  social functions 67–8
  transcultural 95–6
  Victorian era 10–17
Nursing models 152–3

Organisations/institutions
  control by concealment 53–5
  self-interest in 52–3

Patient's Charter 124
Pay, nurses' 108, 118–19
Poland, health needs 168–9
Politics
  concept of 109
  health care 123–4, 127, 160, 165–7
  nurse education 114–17
  and nursing 107–28, 164–8
  participation in 109–10, 127–8,
    164–5, 167–8
Post Registration Education
  and Practice Project (PREPP)
  35
Power
  abuses of 52–3
  pyramids 73–5
  relations 53–4
Project 2000 35, 36–7, 163
  funding 114–16
  political issues 114–17
  Wales 115–16
Public relations 122–3

Racism 91–5, 113–14
Reasoned action, theory of 22, 23
Reflection-in-action 35, 98
Research in nursing 161–2
Role models 150
  influence on attitudes 27, 28, 33–4
  selection 33–4
Role of nurses
  conflicts in 46, 49–50, 57–9,
    62–3, 108
  duality in 49
  effect of institutional concealment
    53–5
  media/public perception of 112–13
  organisational context 59–60, 63
  patient care 45–6, 48, 56–63
  politics and 107
  social 66–8
  socialisation and 43–4
  stereotyping 64–8
  students' perception 88
  subordinate status and 46–52, 58–63,
    66–7, 71–3
Royal College of Nursing 110–11, 117
Russia, health needs 169

Schemas 24
  attitude 24–5
Self-concept 31–2
Self-efficacy 37–8
Self-perception, and attitude
  development 26, 32, 35
Social cognition 30–1
Social conditions 2–4
  education 4
  health reforms 3–4
  nursing 10–17
  social reforms 5
  women in 6–10
Social functions of nursing 67–8
  Social learning 27–8, 66
Socialisation 31–2
  and attitudes/values 32–4, 135
  integration in 34
  moral 69
  occupational 34, 50–1, 87
  professional 34, 43–4, 86, 100
Status of nurses/nursing 46–52, 58–63,
  71–3, 160
  gender and 66–7
Statutory bodies 124–7
Stereotyping
  and attitude development 26
  nurses' role 64–8

sex-role 65–6
Stress, social support 33
Strikes 108, 120
Students
  and assessment 96–8
  bursaries 115, 151
  coping strategies 86–9
  educational resources for 98–9
  interaction with ward staff 87–8
  labelling by teachers 89–90
  relationship with teachers 97
  values 144, 150
Support systems, nurses 33
Support workers, health care *see* health
  care support workers

Teachers
  changing role 36–8
  labelling of students 89–90
  racism 91–5
  relationship with students 97
  use of language 89
Theory, relationship to practice of
  nursing 27, 35–6, 149–55, 162–3
Third World, health needs 169
Timetables, hidden curriculum 84–6
Trade unions 110–11, 117–18
Training of nurses
  Nightingale School 11–12,
    15–16
  otherwise see under education
    of nurses
Transcultural nursing 95–6
Trusts, National Health Service
  123–4

Uniforms 139–43, 161
United Kingdom Central Council
  (UKCC) 124–7
  Code of Conduct 126

Values 23, 131–2
  and attitudes 23–4, 135
  clarification 131–5
  conflict of 136, 137–9
  definitions 22, 23, 131
  hidden agendas 160–2
  hierarchies 135–6
  individual variations 136–7
  institutions 137–8
  nurse education 144–9, 163
  and nursing transgressions
    146–7

objectivity/subjectivity and
    133–4
occupation and 23–4
peculiar to nursing 155–6, 160–1
relationship between personal and
    professional values 132–5

socialisation and 135
student nurses 144, 150, 151
systems 135–6, 137–8
Victorian era 2–17

Women, Victorian 6–10

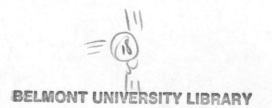

BELMONT UNIVERSITY LIBRARY